A Guide to **SKYLINE DRIVE**
and the **BLUE RIDGE PARKWAY**

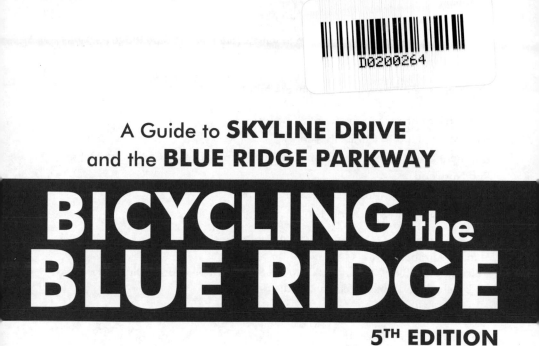

BICYCLING the BLUE RIDGE

5TH EDITION

Elizabeth and
Charlie Skinner

Menasha Ridge Press – Birmingham, Alabama

Bicycling the Blue Ridge: A Guide to Skyline Drive and the Blue Ridge Parkway

5th Edition 2014
Copyright © 2014 by Elizabeth Skinner and Charlie Skinner

Front cover photo © Aurora Photos/Alamy
Back cover photo by Elizabeth Skinner
All interior photos by Elizabeth and Charlie Skinner, Dennis Coello, Bud Zehmer, and Rob Norwood
Cover design and cartography by Scott McGrew
Text design updated by Annie Long

Library of Congress Cataloging-in-Publication Data
Skinner, Elizabeth, 1962–
  Bicycling the Blue Ridge : a guide to the Skyline Drive and the Blue Ridge Parkway / by Elizabeth and Charlie Skinner. – 5th edition.
      pages cm.
  Includes index.
  ISBN-13: 978-0-89732-618-6
  ISBN-10: 0-89732-618-0
 1. Bicycle touring–Virginia–Skyline Drive–Guidebooks. 2. Bicycle touring–Blue Ridge Parkway (N.C. and Va.)–Guidebooks. 3. Skyline Drive (Va.)–Guidebooks. 4. Blue Ridge Parkway (N.C. and Va.)–Guidebooks. I. Skinner, Charlie, 1943– II. Title.
  GV1045.5.V82S626 2014
  796.6'409755–dc23

                         2014005336

ISBN: 978-0-89732-618-6; eISBN: 978-0-89732-951-4

Manufactured in the United States of America

Published by: Menasha Ridge Press
                 c/o Keen Communications
                 PO Box 43673
                 Birmingham, AL 35243
                 800-443-7227
                 info@menasharidge.com
                 menasharidge.com

Visit our website for a complete listing of our books and for ordering information.

Distributed by Publishers Group West

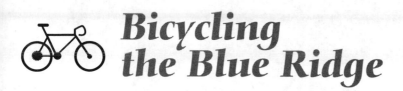

Bicycling
the Blue Ridge

For Bonnie, Caroline, and Katie.

In memory of Willis David Johnson and Rosamond Foltyn.

Table of Contents

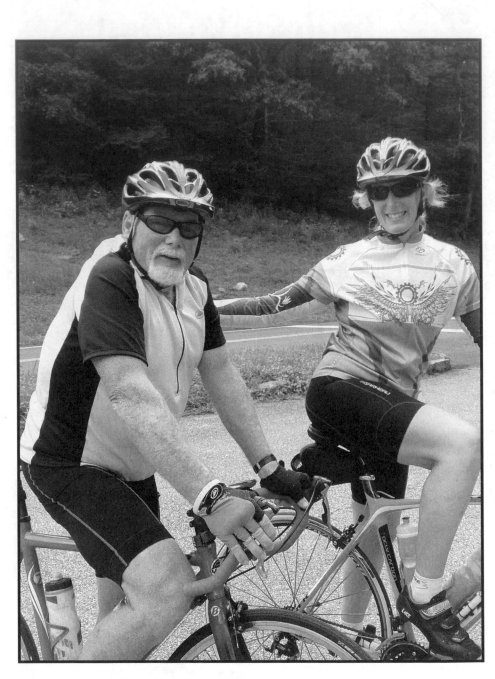

Authors Charlie and Libby Skinner

Acknowledgments

Completing the fifth edition has been a hard-earned process as well as a reclamation of fitness for both Charlie and me after emerging from the demanding years of parenting young children. Unanticipated was Charlie's serious cycling accident and recovery in 2013. Thankfully, Charlie is mended and back on an awesome new bike. In addition to nurturing a deep love of bicycling, I now train and compete in triathlons and have worked to juggle raising two teenage daughters with training for triathlons, researching the book, and keeping up with my job.

There are many people to thank, but we owe the most to our family and bicycling and triathlon friends. You guys know who you are, but a few people must be named. Charlie is forever bonded to Edmund Porter and Jeannie Yingling–all three survived a cycling accident with a 1979 Chevy pickup truck. I am in the best shape of my life due to the coaching guidance of Nick Nothoff and to the support of my swimming, cycling, and triathlon friends Bev Amick, Lynn Bassler, Sara Byerly, Kathy Hardison, John Morris, Miriam Van Patton, Lisa Saunders, Julie Searcy, Celia Sloan, and Jim Williams. The cycling and triathlon community in Winston-Salem is so extensive; thank you to the many folks who have supported Charlie and me along the way.

We would like to thank Ken Putnam, Matt Canter, Charlie Lawrence, and Bob of Ken's Bike Shop for imparting cycling wisdom and for keeping our bikes tuned up and ready to go.

In researching the first edition, Kathleen and Fred Wheeless served as sounding boards for our ideas and provided needed assistance with photography. The original data for the elevation profiles was developed by Jeff Patton, associate professor of geography at the University of North Carolina at Greensboro, and further enhanced by Bud Zehmer, who, on behalf of Menasha Ridge Press, also performed extensive research and editing for the fourth edition. Thanks to Annie Long, whose talent in graphic design brings a crisp look to the interior of the book. Photographs by Elizabeth Skinner and Rob Norwood spruce up the new edition. Thanks to Molly Merkle, Scott McGrew, Susan Roberts McWilliams, and Amber Kaye Henderson for their guidance in the creation of this edition.

Thank you to my closest colleague and friend, Mary McAfee, who has listened to and advised me with compassion, wisdom, and patience for more than 25 years.

As always, we are indebted to our family for their love and support. My deepest gratitude goes to my mom; my sisters, Carole and Jenny; and our awesome and beautiful daughters, Bonnie, Caroline, and Katie.

—Libby Skinner

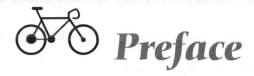 *Preface*

There is no ribbon of highway more ideal for bicycling than Skyline Drive and the Blue Ridge Parkway. Perhaps we feel this way because we stubbornly seek out roads that are enticing to the senses and physically challenging. We spent the greater part of our lives in Florida, a state summed up by bicyclists as hot, flat, and full of headwinds. There is no fall season in Florida; it's pretty much green year-round. So bicycling against a backdrop of yellow, russet, and orange was a new experience for us. Despite our 28 years of exploration by bicycle, the Blue Ridge continues to amaze us.

Now let us concede from the beginning: Skyline Drive and the Blue Ridge Parkway are never easy. You simply cannot be a passive cyclist on these roads. You work excruciatingly hard climbing its mountains, but the descents are more thrilling than your favorite roller coaster ride. They're scarier too, for the controls are all yours. All senses are alert. Body and machine meet rubber and pavement in a high-voltage connection.

Cycling on Skyline Drive and the Blue Ridge Parkway can be a humbling experience. The bicyclist who attempts these roads has definitely signed up for some tough mountain cycling. If the worst hill you've tackled is that bridge or overpass in your otherwise flat hometown, you are in for a big shock. We will address this matter of hill climbing later. First, a word about what motivated us to write this book.

In our travels on Skyline Drive and the Blue Ridge Parkway, we have met cyclists from France, Germany, Japan, California, Florida, and Texas, all in varying stages of bewilderment and frustration. Skyline Drive and the Blue Ridge Parkway present special challenges to the cyclist. In addition to steep road grades, weather conditions are often a menace. Rain, fog, and gusty winds are possible. Facilities are set up for the convenience of the car traveler. Food stops may simply be too far apart to be practical for the bicyclist. Because the National Park Service allows no advertising on Skyline Drive and the Blue Ridge Parkway, motels, restaurants, medical facilities, and the like are often hidden.

Facilities as close as a half mile off the Parkway may be completely concealed from view. Even the literature that outlines facilities off Skyline Drive and the Blue Ridge Parkway is almost exclusively designed for the car traveler. We have learned the hard way about turning off the Parkway only to find ourselves in an immediate descent to nowhere. This means only one thing: a tough climb back up the side of a mountain. And we *like* to climb. If only there were a traveler's guide written for bicyclists from their point of view.

We wrote this book with three groups of bicyclists in mind: racers, long-distance touring cyclists, and recreational cyclists. The Blue Ridge Parkway and Skyline Drive have much to offer each group. Of course, many bicyclists cross over between categories.

Overall, this book is designed for the touring bicyclist who plans to ride Skyline Drive and the Blue Ridge Parkway in an extended tour. In our view, this approach maximizes the experience. However, nothing is more gratifying than a hard ride with just you, your racing bike, and the mountains–no gear, no hassles. We live in Winston-Salem, North Carolina, and a single Sunday ride on the Blue Ridge Parkway can sustain us at least until the next weekend.

If you are a racer, you may not care about campgrounds and motels, but you would probably appreciate knowing where the country stores and other food stops are. We can think of no better training ground for a racer than these roads.

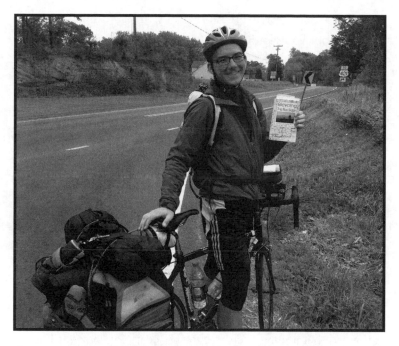

German cyclist headed to the Parkway

New to this edition is a chapter on recommended day and overnight trips. While you may be fortunate enough to be planning an extended tour, the reality is that most of us are looking for a section of the Parkway for a day or weekend trip. All of Skyline Drive and the Parkway make for excellent cycling, but some sections are stellar and should not be missed.

Part of the fun of bicycle touring is making discoveries along the way. We do not want to take any mystery away from this. Our hope is that this book can enhance your experience. As the touring cyclist, you still have the excitement of coming upon the delights of the area, but perhaps you won't find yourself famished because of a 10-mile miscalculation over the next food stop. Little Switzerland is only a half mile from the Parkway, but you would never know of its gastronomic promise as you cruised past Milepost 334.

DISCLAIMER

Bicyclists assume responsibility for their own safety each time they undertake a bicycle trip. No guidebook can alert you to up-to-the-minute changes in weather, traffic, and road conditions. Each cyclist should consider his or her own abilities when planning a bicycle tour of the Blue Ridge. We strongly urge you to wear a helmet.

As of the publication of the fifth edition in 2014, the National Park Service had experienced budget shortfalls and serious closures along the Blue Ridge Parkway. Parkway administration could not predict when some facilities would reopen, if at all. It is estimated that it may take three to five years for some facilities to reopen. For up-to-date facility closures, visit the Blue Ridge Parkway website at **nps.gov/blri** or call the information line at 828-298-0398.

The National Park Service has also struggled to maintain road surfaces along the Blue Ridge Parkway. There is a 10–15 year maintenance schedule for resurfacing the Parkway, but it would seem that there is always at least one section of 5–20 miles that is in a state of disrepair with potholes and crumbling asphalt. Rockslides and adverse weather conditions can also erode road surfaces. Just be aware that you may encounter a pothole here and there.

May all your cycling adventures be safe and full of fun, thrills, and excitement.

PART 1
An Introduction to Bicycling the Blue Ridge

The Ultimate Bicycling Road

For the bicyclist, the Blue Ridge Parkway and Skyline Drive present an impressive list of statistics. Combined, these two highways comprise 575 miles of continuous road, which rides the crest of the Blue Ridge Mountains. The Blue Ridge Mountains are the eastern rampart of the Appalachian Mountains extending from southern Pennsylvania to northern Georgia. Skyline Drive and the Blue Ridge Parkway enable the bicyclist to experience a large portion of the Blue Ridge Mountains. These two roads can transport you from Front Royal, Virginia (just 67 miles from Washington, D.C.), to Cherokee in the southwest corner of North Carolina at the gateway of the Great Smoky Mountains National Park. Skyline Drive extends 105 miles from Front Royal to Rockfish Gap just outside Waynesboro, Virginia. At Rockfish Gap the road continues uninterrupted as the Blue Ridge Parkway.

Although elevations in the Blue Ridge are modest compared to the Rockies or the Sierra Nevada, changes in elevation on Skyline Drive and the Parkway are fairly irregular. The highest elevation on Skyline Drive and the Blue Ridge Parkway (hereafter referred to as the Parkway) is 6,053 feet at Richland Balsam in the Great Balsams between Mount Pisgah and Cherokee. The next highest elevations are in the Black Mountain range, which is in the southernmost section of the Parkway. One of the most exhilarating side trips off either road is the 5-mile climb to the summit of Mount Mitchell, which at 6,684 feet is the highest point in the eastern United States. The lowest point of the roads is near Otter Creek in Virginia, at 649 feet.

After many talks with bicyclists on the Parkway and Skyline Drive, we think that it is fair to say that changes in elevation are a major preoccupation with bicyclists who undertake the Blue Ridge. If we have learned nothing else in our thousands of miles logged on the Parkway and Skyline Drive, it is that cycling is much more enjoyable if you can somehow manage to suspend all worry about elevation and just take it as it comes. Conceding that elevation is critical to cyclists, we have detailed changes in elevation in our point-by-point descriptive section.

The Blue Ridge Mountains have a rich geologic history. As a part of the Appalachian mountain range, the Blue Ridge Mountains are among the oldest mountains on Earth. As you cycle past sheer granite walls, some blasted through in the construction of these roads, think about the amount of time Precambrian rock represents: the geologic upheaval that formed the Appalachian mountain range took place about 200 million years ago during the Paleozoic era.

For bicyclists, wind is often the dominant element dictating the pace and the effort required to travel from point A to point B. The wind has smoothed and carved the Blue Ridge over millions of years. Angles here are not severe and jagged like in the Rockies, but windswept and misty with mosses, wildflowers, balsams, rhododendrons, and mountain laurels that seem to ease the mountain back to earth. Edward Abbey brings the geologic history of the Appalachians to its logical conclusion in *Appalachian Wilderness:*

> *What the future holds for the mountains, according to geology, is simply a long continuation of the present erosional downgrading which will end, presumably, given enough time and if the world lasts that long, with the Appalachians as we know them reduced to a more or less featureless peneplain—to no more, that is, than a gently rolling surface of rock and field and forest (we hope) not much above sea level.*

We are lucky to have these mountains here in the South. People gravitate to the timelessness and calm of the Blue Ridge for renewal and refuge. Interestingly, Great Smoky Mountains National Park is the most heavily visited park in the National Park System.

History chronicles the people who settled in the Blue Ridge before any talk of national parks. Many of these people were of Scotch-Irish descent, and other settlers were German immigrants from the Black Forest, who introduced techniques for building cabins like those of their homeland. All who persisted and survived the rugged conditions and isolation of the Blue Ridge surmounted many obstacles. The folklore and specialized knowledge these mountain people possessed are now celebrated as a unique and important heritage.

Opportunities for reflection on the culture of the Blue Ridge are readily available along Skyline Drive and the Parkway. The National Park Service (NPS) has designed displays, signs, and visitor centers to illustrate the lifestyle of the early settlers. Several sites demonstrate the daily life of the mountain culture. The working farm at Humpback Rocks Visitor Center is run by

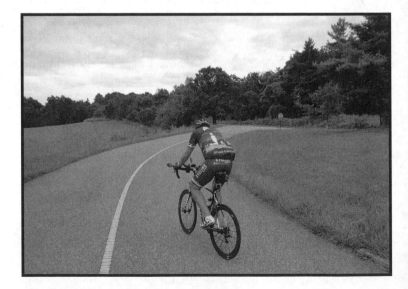

Heading onto the Parkway from an overlook

NPS staff who dress in period costume and tend the farm using early methods. The gristmill at Mabry Mill operates year-round: there is no better place to see authentic apparatus used to make sorghum, molasses, and apple butter during the fall season. Caudill Cabin, visible in the Doughton Park area, invites the traveler to speculate on the isolation of existence in the Blue Ridge. The Blue Ridge Music Center near Fancy Gap, Virginia, features extensive exhibits on the history of music traditions of the area and hosts bluegrass and mountain music concerts nearly every weekend May–October.

Anyone who spends even a week bicycle-touring the Blue Ridge can experience a hint of the vulnerability that early settlers encountered in this unyielding, sparsely populated area. Although the mountains are becoming increasingly developed in tourist areas, the Parkway and Skyline Drive continue to remain uncluttered by modern conveniences such as fast-food restaurants and mini-malls. For those, the Blue Ridge still requires us to descend from its peaks, however narrow national park boundaries may be.

On the other hand, the Moses H. Cone Memorial Park and Mount Pisgah provide a glimpse into the wealth of the famous industrialists, Moses H. Cone and George Vanderbilt, both of whom built lavish mountain retreats. The contrast has always been great between subsistence farmers whose livelihood depends on the mountains and tourists who come to the Blue Ridge for sport and leisure.

The history of the construction of Skyline Drive and the Parkway is rife with controversy. A number of proposed routes were mapped out before settling on the present one. The state of Tennessee campaigned heavily to host the Parkway but ultimately lost out to North Carolina. The visionary behind a road that would connect Shenandoah National Park to Great Smoky Mountains National Park is said to have been Virginia senator

Harry F. Byrd. However, Theodore E. Straus, who was a public works administrator from Maryland, is also credited as the originator of the idea.

Officially, Franklin D. Roosevelt, Congress, the Virginia State Legislature, the people of Virginia and North Carolina, and the NPS were responsible for following through with the project. Skyline Drive was begun through an Act of Congress. Due to the stipulation that no federal money be spent to acquire land for Skyline Drive, the Virginia State Legislature appropriated more than a million dollars and then solicited the people of Virginia to donate land and matching funds. The Civilian Conservation Corps completed Skyline Drive in 1939.

President Roosevelt was so pleased by the success of Skyline Drive that he approved a joint project by the NPS and the Bureau of Public Roads to connect Shenandoah National Park with Great Smoky Mountains National Park. The Blue Ridge Parkway was not officially completed until 1987 with the opening of the Linn Cove Viaduct. Before its completion travelers had to take a brief detour in the Boone–Blowing Rock area to circumvent privately owned Grandfather Mountain.

Although the Linn Cove Viaduct is celebrated as an engineering marvel, the entire Skyline Drive and Parkway project is masterful. It is astounding that so many diverse groups of people came together to build the mountain highway: politicians who were immersed in their agendas, government officials who oversaw the project, highway engineers and landscape architects who were focused on the path of the road, mountain folk who were employed by the Civilian Conservation Corps during the Depression, skilled artisans from Europe who crafted the elegant stone bridges and tunnels, landowners who were coaxed into selling their land, and naturalists who were concerned with the environmental impact of the road.

Because this book champions what the Parkway and Skyline Drive have to offer bicyclists, we should point out four simple facts that make these roads ideal for our mode of travel. There are no route changes with which to contend; the road surface is well above average; commercial traffic is prohibited; and the speed limit is much lower than that of a regular highway.

There are no route changes. Skyline Drive makes a seamless transition into the Blue Ridge Parkway at Rockfish Gap, Virginia. If you are traveling north, you will be required to pay a small fee upon entering Skyline Drive from the Parkway. Skyline Drive is a toll road, and fees are collected at all entrance stations. This entitles you to seven days of travel along Skyline Drive.

From time to time, we have been disoriented regarding whether to head north or south when driving or cycling up onto the Parkway from an entrance ramp. When you enter at random from a highway that intersects the Parkway, you encounter a sign that states simply **BLUE RIDGE PARKWAY** (with arrows pointing north or south). You must proceed in one direction in order to find a sign that states a destination and its mileage. Skyline Drive has four designated entry points: Front Royal, Virginia, the northernmost entry point; followed by Thornton Gap; Swift Run Gap; and Rockfish Gap. Signage is very clear at all of these points.

The road surface on both highways is generally good. However, conditions do change with time. For example, during one season the NPS upgraded much of the drainage system and some of the overlooks along Skyline Drive. This meant several construction sites that caused traffic to be routed onto a single lane. The Twin Tunnels were being repaired on the Parkway. The NPS was also doing major roadwork between Asheville and Mount Pisgah. These are all situations where the NPS was in the process of maintaining and upgrading the road. From 2012 to 2014 the NPS has struggled to resurface the Parkway section by section. At any given time, it is possible to encounter potholes and deteriorating road conditions in brief sections.

If you are concerned about problems with road conditions, we suggest that you call ahead of time for a current report on ongoing construction. For conditions along Skyline Drive, call for information at 540-999-3500; along the Parkway, call 828-298-0398. You can visit the Blue Ridge website, **nps.gov/blri.** You can also ask a park ranger upon arrival at either park. For emergencies, call 800-732-0911.

Although the NPS actively maintains these roads, weather and erosion can create temporary problems and wash out sections of the road. Fallen rocks, broken limbs or fallen trees, dead animals, and roads slick with rain or ice are potential hazards. The NPS has

Stone mileposts are positioned at each mile on both Skyline Drive and the Blue Ridge Parkway.

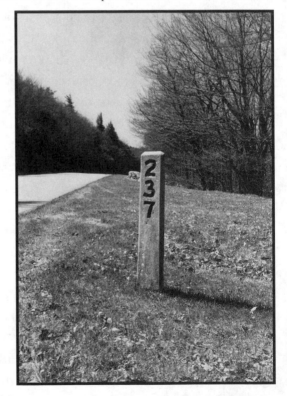

posted signs in falling rock zones. You will also find warning signs for deer crossings and signs announcing all tunnels.

Both roads are clearly marked with signs denoting overlooks, campgrounds, picnic areas, ranger stations, intersecting highways, elevation points, hiking trails, and any other facilities sponsored by the NPS. The NPS prohibits all advertising along these roads. Some enterprising business people perch signs on hillsides beyond park boundaries, hopeful that travelers will spot them as they gaze at the countryside. In many cases, country stores and motels go unnoticed even though they are less than a mile from the road.

One sign that carries great significance for bicyclists is the milepost marker. Stone mileposts are positioned at each mile on both Skyline Drive and the Parkway. Just as you can get hung up on elevation, anticipating every mile is no fun either. They are hard to miss, though. Most of us probably register every single marker subconsciously, and they are indispensable in charting your way through the Blue Ridge. It's not likely that you will ever get lost on Skyline Drive or the Parkway.

There is no paved shoulder or bicycle lane on either road, but we have never felt this to be a great loss. The road is amply wide enough for a car and a bike. The only vehicles that some-times cause problems are RVs and their drivers who sometimes underestimate the size of their vehicles on the road.

Also, beware of wide mirrors on pickups or vehicles towing campers. The full length of some people's camping entourage is amazing and, from a bicyclist's perspective, insane. It is common to see a full-size pickup truck pulling not only an Airstream camper but also a car for sightseeing–the total camping unit. As horrific as this sounds, we can deal with it when we consider that the maximum speed limit on Skyline Drive is 35 miles per hour and only 45 miles per hour on the Parkway. Do keep in mind that *scenic highway* implies tourist traffic. The majority of travelers on these roads are there to sightsee. Drivers are not always paying attention to their driving. Cars occasionally come to abrupt stops or suddenly pull off the road: erratic behavior is common.

Never having to worry about commercial truck traffic is a major advantage that Skyline Drive and the Parkway offer bicyclists. We all cope with adverse conditions on unrestricted roads, so not having to worry about 10 tons of steel looming from behind is very liberating. Even if you are highly selective about the roads you cycle, a highway that prohibits commercial traffic is rare. You may encounter occasional delivery trucks headed for one of the National Park Service concessions, but they take the most expedient routes on and off these roads.

There are two primary differences between Skyline Drive and the Blue Ridge Parkway. Skyline Drive is a toll road, and elevations on Skyline Drive do not reach the extremes of those on the Parkway. The highest point on Skyline Drive is 3,680 feet. Generally, Skyline Drive rides a plateau. Once you have climbed up to the 3,000-foot range, you will find markedly less variation in elevation than on the Parkway until you descend at either end. By comparison, the Parkway has wild variations in elevation. In a 30-mile stretch from Otter Creek to the Peaks of Otter, you cycle from the lowest point on the Parkway in Virginia at 649 feet to the highest point on the Parkway in Virginia at 3,950 feet.

One other difference between Skyline Drive and the Parkway is the number of NPS concessions. Skyline Drive has an abundance of restaurants, campgrounds, and lodges well spaced for bicyclists. The Parkway is less consistent: NPS concessions are as close together as 35 miles and as far apart as 70 miles. Careful planning is not only smart but also necessary.

The NPS has put some thought into the reality of bicyclists and motorists coexisting on the Parkway and Skyline Drive by announcing in their literature and signage the necessity that

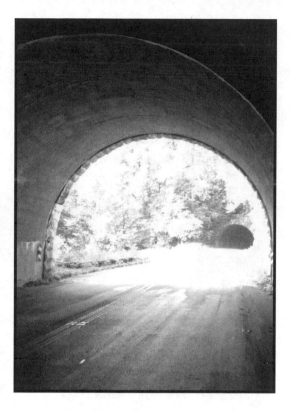

*2 of the 27 tunnels
on the Parkway*

motorists be alert to bicyclists. For example, bicycle-warning signs are present at the opening of each of the 27 tunnels on the Parkway and the single tunnel on Skyline Drive.

Visibility in these tunnels is cause for concern and should be taken seriously. None of the tunnels have artificial lighting, so the longer tunnels are pitch-black inside. Even when using lights we have felt out of control in some tunnels, especially those south of Waterrock Knob near Cherokee. The descent in this area ranges from 5,718 feet to 2,020 feet. Just imagine entering these tunnels from bright sunshine at speeds between 30 and 45 miles per hour. Suddenly, you've lost the edge of the road and everything is black. You're still seeing the afterglow of the sun. Next, you hear something large and heavy rumbling up ahead. It's probably an

RV. You're getting very unsure of yourself very fast. In the section on equipment, we discuss how to prepare for tunnels.

We feel that bicyclists could command greater respect for their rights if they did their part to share the road with cars. In fact, the NPS has published guidelines and warnings about road conditions for bicyclists.

BICYCLING REGULATIONS

* Bicycle riders must comply with all applicable state and federal motor vehicle regulations.
* Bicycles may be ridden only on paved road surfaces and parking areas. Bicycles, including mountain bikes, may not be ridden on trails or walkways.
* The bicycle operator must exhibit a white light or reflector visible at least 500 feet to the front and a red light or reflector visible at least 200 feet to the rear during periods of low visibility between the hours of sunset and sunrise, or while traveling through a tunnel.
* Bicycles must be ridden single file (except when passing or turning left) and well to the right-hand side of the road.
* Bicycle speed must be reasonable for control with regard to traffic, weather, road, and light conditions.

FOR SAFE BICYCLING

* Wear a bicycle helmet.
* Be sure your bicycle is in good operating condition. Carry a spare tube and tools for minor repairs.
* Wear high-visibility clothing. It sets you apart from the scenery and makes you more noticeable to motorists.
* Avoid the Parkway during periods of low visibility. Fog and rain may occur unpredictably. Reschedule your trip for better weather or follow lower elevation routes until weather conditions improve.

* Exercise caution when riding through tunnels. Be sure your bicycle is equipped with proper lights or reflectors. There are 26 tunnels in North Carolina and 1 tunnel in Virginia.
* Temperatures vary greatly along the Parkway due to different elevations. Wear your clothing in layers.
* Safe drinking water is available at all picnic areas, camp-grounds, concession operations, and visitor centers. Water from streams and springs is unsafe for drinking unless you purify it.
* Make an honest evaluation of your abilities before beginning a bicycle trip on the Parkway. In some sections, you will climb as much as 1,100 feet in 3.4 miles.
* When cycling in a group, adjust your spacing to allow motor vehicles to pass safely.

EXTENDED TRIPS

* Some Parkway campgrounds and services are located too far apart for convenient cycling.
* Camping is permitted only at established campgrounds. In some areas, the U.S. Forest Service, state parks, and private campgrounds are within easy distance of the Parkway. However, many operate on a seasonal basis.
* Food and lodging services are also available along and adjacent to the Parkway. Most operate seasonally.
* To assist in planning your trip, consult the Parkway Map and Blue Ridge Parkway Directory.
* Carry a simple first-aid kit.
* Contact a ranger before leaving a motor vehicle parked overnight on the Parkway.

We think these guidelines are reasonable. Just remember how privileged we are to have such a road along the Blue Ridge. If you live for the ultimate road, this is it.

Weather in the Blue Ridge Mountains

Weather in the Blue Ridge Mountains has amazing, beautiful contrasts. Each season highlights special characteristics of the mountains. Bicycling in the southern Appalachians is great during much of the year, as long as you know what to expect and prepare with the proper clothing. Weather can make or break a cycling trip in the Blue Ridge. That is true in any bicycling situation, but even more so in the mountains, where weather fronts can move in suddenly, making weather a major consideration. Call 828-298-0398 for up-to-date closures and weather-related info.

The Blue Ridge is famous for its display of fall colors. During autumn expect near bumper-to-bumper traffic, especially on the northern half of Skyline Drive, which draws hordes of leaf peepers from the nearby Washington area. This is the biggest tourist time of the year. If you dislike competing with cars for your share of the road, we suggest that you avoid weekends during peak leaf time.

Then November suddenly arrives with its wind and rain, which render the trees bare, and few care about the Blue Ridge except its true-blue aficionados. Houses usually hidden deep in the woods are revealed. Ridges and other physical features of the mountains rise in relief. Fall days on the Parkway can be crisp and bright or overcast with a somber, damp chill that has you preferring a cozy fire to a brisk ride.

Winter is perhaps the most difficult season for the bicyclist, but it can be thrilling. December–February (and sometimes into March), the Parkway may be best suited for cross-country skiing. Winter is certainly the most brutal season; the gnarled, stunted trees are a testament to winter's harsh winds. Snow and ice are treacherous. The National Park Service (NPS) closes off some sections of the road with gates barring car traffic.

Ice is the most serious hazard. We recommend mountain bikes in the winter months. You can find steel-studded mountain bike tires for riding in snow and ice. Extended touring in the winter is not advised; day trips are more practical. Not only is the road difficult, but open facilities are scarce November 1–May 1. Just make sure that you plan carefully and know the weather forecast before you venture out. Selected NPS campgrounds are winterized and are open all winter.

Spring never seems to come soon enough for cyclists who have had to cope with bitter winter temperatures. This is aggravated by the spring's reputation for unpredictability. Even though it is officially spring on the calendar, the Blue Ridge may be destined for more weeks of bitter temperatures. During a recent March, we experienced a glorious weekend of cobalt-blue skies when T-shirts and cycling shorts were the only clothing we required. The next weekend the temperature dropped 30 degrees, but we thought we could handle it. We had balaclavas, tights, polypropylene, and wind jackets, and we were truly miserable. The wind was devastating. If you drive up from the Piedmont or other lower elevations, remember that the mountains can easily be 10 degrees cooler.

There is usually less rain in the spring. Although we cyclists can do without rain, lack of rain in the spring months can cause serious drought conditions in the Blue Ridge. Planning a cycling trip on the Blue Ridge in early spring is risky. You really need to keep a close eye on the weather forecast and know your tolerance level. Good weather or bad, the greatest challenge for many cyclists in the spring is getting back in top form and toughing out the longer ascents.

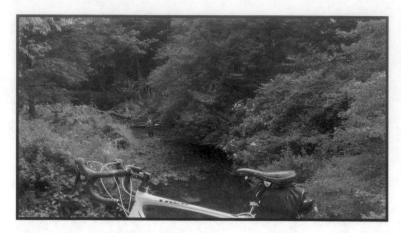

Taking a break to watch a fly fisherman below

Summer is the premier cycling season. Temperatures are warm, the foliage is lush and green, and wildflowers and rhododendrons provide bright contrasts in color. When summer finally comes, it is a great feeling to shed all of those winter layers and cycle unencumbered by weight and bulk.

Summer in the Blue Ridge can be hot and humid; it can also be wet with sudden thunderstorms and fog. According to National Climatic Data Center statistics, the summer months are the foggiest of the year. In June, July, and August, there are an average of 11 days each month with less than a quarter-mile visibility due to heavy fog. August ranks highest with an average of 14 days of heavy fog; September comes in second with 12 days. Fog really can force you off the Parkway and Skyline Drive. We always tour with a flashing belt beacon for the rear of our bikes and a white light for the front. Visibility can be practically nil. The odds are high of encountering at least one morning or afternoon of inclement weather in a week's trip.

To illustrate the frustrations that weather can cause cyclists, we would like to talk about September. We chose September twice in the past four years for extended cycling trips. One reason was that September, statistically, does not rank among the rainiest months in the Blue Ridge. The mean number of days with one-tenth of an inch or more of precipitation is eight. Eight to 30, those odds don't sound too bad.

The first time we toured the entire length of Skyline Drive and the Parkway, we experienced rain and fog every day for two weeks, from Front Royal, Virginia, to Blowing Rock, North Carolina. On our second September tour, the last 36 hours were a total rainout. The moral of the story: Weather in the Blue Ridge is unpredictable, so prepare for its downside. If you cannot handle cycling through rain, you will definitely need to factor a few extra days into your travel itinerary.

One final aspect of the weather that you should be aware of is wind. Headwinds are never much of a problem in the mountains. The surprise for those who have never cycled in the mountains is wind gusting through gaps. Most gaps are labeled by signs along Skyline Drive and the Parkway. In his *Blue Ridge Parkway Guide*, William G. Lord calls upon mountain folklore to define a gap:

> *See the outline of that mountain over thar? Them low dips in it's what's knowed as a gap. Some of 'm is whar a road or trail is located acrost the mountains.*

In general, the Parkway travels the crest line of the Blue Ridge and several other ranges. Therefore, it passes through a long series of gaps and intersects many cross-mountain roads.

On a windy day, gusts of wind may blow through these gaps in a mountain. You can be shooting down the side of a mountain only to find yourself fighting for control of your bike. A firm grip on the handlebars and confident bike-handling skills should prevent any mishaps.

On the following pages, we have compiled data on temperature and precipitation available from the National Climatic Data Center in Asheville, North Carolina.

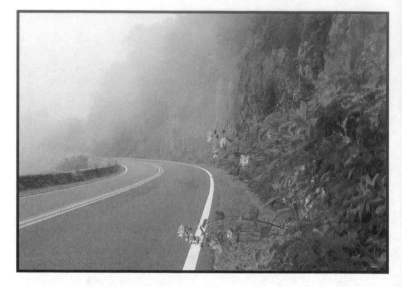

Fog rolls in and visibility becomes a problem.

AVERAGE DAILY MAXIMUM AND MINIMUM TEMPERATURES (°F)									
	Asheville		Boone		Roanoke		Peaks of Otter		Big Meadows	
	HI	LO	HI	LO	HI	LO	HI	LO	HI	LO
JAN	47	26	44	25	45	26	na		na	
FEB	51	28	46	25	48	28	na		na	
MAR	58	34	52	31	57	35	na	43	na	37
APR	69	43	62	38	68	44	64	52	59	46
MAY	76	51	71	47	76	53	72	58	67	54
JUN	81	51	77	55	83	60	77	53	74	57
JUL	84	62	79	59	87	65	81	52	76	56
AUG	83	62	79	58	85	64	79	56	75	50
SEP	78	56	73	51	79	57	73	46	69	na
OCT	69	43	65	41	69	45	63	46	60	na
NOV	59	34	53	32	67	36	na		na	
DEC	50	28	44	25	48	29	na		na	

AVERAGE MONTHLY PRECIPITATION IN INCHES				
	Asheville	Boone	Roanoke	Peaks of Otter	Big Meadows
JAN	3.48"	4.05"	2.83"	na	na
FEB	3.60"	4.08"	3.19"	na	na
MAR	5.13"	5.14"	3.69"	na	na
APR	3.84"	4.45"	3.09"	na	na
MAY	4.19"	4.34"	3.51"	na	na
JUN	4.20"	4.52"	3.34"	na	na
JUL	4.43"	5.94"	3.45"	na	na
AUG	4.79"	5.33"	3.91"	5.50"	5.47"
SEP	3.96"	4.40"	3.14"	na	na
OCT	3.29"	3.16"	3.48"	3.51"	na
NOV	3.29"	4.34"	3.94"	na	na
DEC	3.51"	2.59"	2.93"	na	na

MEAN NUMBER OF DAYS WITH 0.01 INCH OR MORE OF PRECIPITATION			
	Asheville	Boone*	Roanoke
JAN	10 days	9 days	10 days
FEB	9 days	7 days	10 days
MAR	11 days	9 days	11 days
APR	9 days	8 days	10 days
MAY	12 days	8 days	12 days
JUN	11 days	9 days	10 days
JUL	12 days	11 days	12 days
AUG	12 days	9 days	11 days
SEP	9 days	7 days	8 days
OCT	8 days	5 days	8 days
NOV	9 days	6 days	9 days
DEC	10 days	7 days	9 days

* 0.1 inch or more

Camping versus Lodging

If you are considering an extended tour of Skyline Drive and the Parkway, the first decision you will probably make is whether to camp or stay in motels. There are pros and cons to both approaches. However, if you can afford motels, your trip will be easier and more comfortable. Without a sleeping bag, pad, tent, and cooking gear, you can make better time on the road. Credit-card touring is definitely the streamlined way to go.

Many lodges along Skyline Drive and the Parkway are memorable for their high ceilings and exposed beams, large stone fireplaces, decks and porches for lounging, and restaurants featuring southern mountain cooking. From people-watching by the fireplace in the great room at Big Meadows to gazing out at the lights of Asheville from the deck of Pisgah Inn, lodges heighten the rustic mountain experience.

There are five lodges within strict National Park Service (NPS) boundaries of Skyline Drive and the Parkway. Although Skyland Resort and Big Meadows Lodge are spaced nicely along Skyline Drive, the lodges along the Parkway are far apart. Peaks of Otter Lodge is 150 miles from Bluffs Lodge at Doughton Park. After that, the only other NPS lodge is at Mount Pisgah. In Part 2 of the book, we outline all NPS and private facilities along these roads.

We have devised a rating system for the cost of motels and lodges. These rates are per night and are subject to change, particularly during special events and during the leaf season. Please call ahead.

$	inexpensive	up to $75
$$	moderate	$75–$125
$$$	expensive	$125 and up

Private concessionaires operate all of the restaurants and lodges along Skyline Drive and the Parkway. There are no other businesses within the boundaries of either park. Essentially, the Blue Ridge Parkway boundaries are very narrow as the road winds through the Blue Ridge. The major facilities along the Parkway include Otter Creek, Peaks of Otter, Roanoke Mountain, Rocky Knob, Mabry Mill, Cumberland Knob, Doughton Park, Moses H. Cone, Julian Price Memorial Park, Linville Falls, Crabtree Meadows, Craggy Gardens, and Mount Pisgah. Skyline Drive differs because it is surrounded by the much larger Shenandoah National Park. While the NPS maintains facilities at Mathews Arm, Skyland, Big Meadows, Lewis Mountain, and Loft Mountain, the surrounding areas along Skyline Drive are protected as national parklands.

Because the Parkway has so few facilities within its boundaries in proportion to its length, we have provided information on motels and campgrounds off the Parkway. When you study the Parkway map, you see that it is feasible to tour from one NPS campground to another. There are some long, difficult stretches between these campgrounds. It is 70 miles from Rocky Knob Campground to Doughton Park Campground, and 65 miles from Doughton Park to the next NPS campground at Julian Price. That may be more than you want to cover in a day. And if it rains or fog sets in, what then? That's why you need alternatives when touring the Parkway. Things hardly ever go according to plan.

NPS campgrounds are distinctive in several ways. They are all situated within large tracts of NPS land ranging in size from 250 acres to 7,000 acres. Most of these campgrounds are fairly secluded in wooded areas, and each has a charm all its own. Otter Creek has its namesake flowing alongside campsites; Peaks of Otter and Julian Price are situated beside lakes; deer roam freely throughout Big Meadows; and you pitch your tent amid gnarled, ancient balsams at Mount Pisgah. Big Meadows on Skyline Drive is the largest campground, with 217 sites. The smallest, Lewis Mountain Campground, has 31 sites and is also on Skyline Drive.

The big difference between Skyline Drive and the Parkway campgrounds is that nearly all Skyline Drive campgrounds have pay showers (the exception is Mathews Arm). There are no showers in Blue Ridge Parkway campgrounds, with the exception of Mount Pisgah. Shenandoah National Park (Skyline Drive) has more conveniences than the Parkway. The camp stores are much more elaborate. The campgrounds along Skyline Drive have laundry facilities. Although several private campgrounds along the Parkway have shower and laundry facilities, none of the NPS campgrounds on the Parkway have either convenience. Most likely, backpackers on the Appalachian Trail are the reason for these amenities on Skyline Drive. With the Appalachian Trail running through Shenandoah National Park and paralleling Skyline Drive, NPS facilities are the primary source for hikers. The Appalachian Trail intersects the Parkway at a few points, but these intersections are not near NPS facilities.

The physical layout of the typical campground in both parks is very similar. Paved roads run through the campgrounds. Tents and RVs have separate areas. Each tent site has a groomed tent pad, picnic table, and grill. Within clustered sites you will find running water, restrooms, and trash receptacles. Some campgrounds have bear poles if the campground is located in bear country. All campgrounds have an amphitheater or gathering place, pay telephones, and rangers on duty.

Daily rates for Skyline Drive campgrounds are $16 per site ($20 per site at Big Meadows after May 13). The Parkway charges $15–$20 per site in all campgrounds. All campgrounds are filled on a first-come, first-serve basis except Big Meadows, which requires reservations. Call 877-444-6777 to place a reservation. Big Meadows remains open through November; the other campgrounds in the park close October 31.

We think that camping is a great experience in and of itself. Although it does require more effort in the long run, combining camping with lodging allows you the best of both worlds. A fully loaded touring bike gives you all the options. If you decide you can go no farther, but there is nothing civilized for miles, you can pull off the road and have a tent over your head and the means to cook a decent meal. With credit-card touring you must plan ahead. If you are not capable of covering the mileage to make your motel reservation, there is little to fall back on.

The best way to decide which approach to bicycle touring suits you is to weigh the pros and cons. We figure it can't hurt to spell them all out.

Camping

ADVANTAGES OF CAMPING:

✳ Camping is less expensive.

✳ Camping is an experience in and of itself.

✳ There is a tendency to meet more people. Campers seem to open up to the novelty of the touring cyclist.

✳ You have more options. With facilities sometimes far apart, it is a plus to have both camping and lodging possibilities.

DISADVANTAGES OF CAMPING:

✳ The extra gear required increases the weight you must carry.

✳ Housekeeping chores, such as setting up and breaking camp, require more time.

✳ There are no showers in Parkway campgrounds with Mount Pisgah being the exception.

✳ You must be prepared for inclement weather.

✳ During peak times, some campgrounds fill up. The campgrounds on Skyline Drive reach capacity more often than those on the Parkway. It can be impossible to obtain sites at peak times. If camping at Big Meadows on Skyline Drive, you must make reservations ahead of time (see page 44).

✱ Only one NPS campground is open in the winter months: Linville Falls in North Carolina (Milepost 316). Most NPS campgrounds open between early April and mid-May and close around October 31 (except for Big Meadows, which is open mid-May until the end of November, and Linville Falls, which is open year-round).

Lodging

ADVANTAGES OF LODGING:

✱ Spending your nights in motels allows streamlined, efficient touring: no sleeping bags, tents, cooking gear, and so on.

✱ With less weight you can tour faster and cover more miles each day.

✱ Some wonderful lodges can be found along Skyline Drive and the Parkway.

✱ You can expect the creature comforts of home: showers; a warm, dry bed; a TV; and so on.

DISADVANTAGES OF LODGING:

✱ Reservations are advisable and, at peak times, required.

✱ Most motels have required check-in times. If you fail to arrive on time at your destination, you may lose your room. Usually, you can guarantee a room with a major credit card.

✱ Motels and lodges are open seasonally. Generally, this is May 1–October 31.

✱ Rates are subject to change.

Gearing Up:
Special Equipment and Clothing

When making choices regarding equipment and clothing for bicycling in the mountains, three tenets should be foremost in your mind:

* Know your abilities.
* Know your bicycle.
* Anticipate the weather.

Everything we say here may seem obvious, but we want to emphasize the key issues.

Bicycles and Tools

With the many choices of high-tech bicycles and cycling equipment on the market, we suggest that you select the best you can afford. If you cannot purchase everything you need all at once, upgrade later. We highly recommend using sealed components as much as possible: sealed headsets, bottom brackets, hubs, and pedals. In the long run, sealed components will endure, especially through adverse weather conditions.

While we choose not to discuss gear ratios, we advise you to make an honest assessment of your abilities when setting your bike up for mountain cycling. The Assault on Mount Mitchell, a 102-mile endurance event, is an extreme case, but it is a classic example of bicyclists getting in over their heads. Each year that we participate, we see a steady procession of cyclists reduced to walking their bikes along the Parkway and the 5 miles up to the summit of Mount Mitchell. This is not the sad fate of one or two cyclists; what you see are 30 or 40 people who thought they would be able to cycle through exhaustion with the gearing they had selected. For more information on the Assault on Mount Mitchell, see the descriptive section on page 103.

If you are considering an extended trip of the Parkway and Skyline Drive, and you have never toured in mountainous terrain, a triple crank set is a must. Fully loaded panniers make a difference in any terrain. Mountains truly magnify any weight you choose to carry.

Having the right tool for the right emergency is not always possible. You should carry the bare essentials on every ride. There are so few bike shops along Skyline Drive and the Parkway that you really need to put some thought into tool selection. If you are day-tripping, it is a good idea to have at least a comprehensive selection of tools in your car and a basic tool kit on your bike. If you are making an extended tour, you want to strike a balance. The weight of tools can really add up, but a bike emergency can leave you stranded. In some situations you may have to hitch a ride to the nearest bike shop. See Appendix A for a list of the bike shops within a reasonable distance of the Parkway.

If you need help selecting tools and equipment for your bike, we suggest that you take your bike to your local shop and ask a mechanic for advice. All good bike shops are more than happy to spend time showing you how to use the proper tools to make minor adjustments on your bike. Of course, any time you cycle on the Parkway, you should make sure that your bike is in top condition.

One investment you might consider is high-quality wheels. Hand-built wheels with sealed hubs should spare you much aggravation. In any event, tools you will want on hand if you are touring are a spoke wrench and spare spokes.

We have compiled a list of the tools we think are absolutely essential. Most of these tools will fit in the type of bag that mounts under a bicycle saddle. If you are making day trips, you can leave off the spokes, cables, and spare tire.

CHARLIE'S LIST OF ESSENTIAL TOOLS

* Chain breaker
* Spoke wrench
* Spare spokes
* Pliers
* Small adjustable wrench
* Allen wrenches
* Tire levers
* Brake cable (front and rear)
* Derailleur cable (front and rear)
* Spare tire, tubes, and patch kit
* Multipurpose lubricant
* Air pump (which attaches to bike frame)

Make sure that your air pump works properly and has the correct head for the type of tube you use, Presta or Schrader. Just remember, on the Parkway and Skyline Drive proper, there is practically zero availability of bicycle parts. A rudimentary knowledge of bicycle repair is a required bicycle skill.

If you have absolutely no mechanical aptitude, you might want to carry a small repair manual that can guide you through basic repairs. After all, compared to most machines, a bicycle is not that complicated. We recommend the following titles:

Linnard Zinn, *Zinn and the Art of Road Bike Maintenance* (Velo Press, 2000)

Rob Van der Plas, *Road Bike Maintenance* (Van der Plas Publications, 1996)

Jim Langley, *Bicycling Magazine's Complete Guide to Bicycle Maintenance and Repair for Road and Mountain Bikes* (Rodale Press, 1999)

CLOTHING

Certain clothing items are essential, even for weekend trips in the Blue Ridge. Needless to say, weather should govern all the clothing choices you make. We highly recommend a Gore-Tex jacket or rainsuit. In our opinion, this item above all others is the most essential for cycling in the Blue Ridge. At the very minimum, a Windbreaker or some water-repellent jacket is a must. This is necessary not only for rain but for sudden cold temperatures and windy conditions as well.

Is Gore-Tex fabric really worth it? We think so. We cycled in the rain with regular nylon rainsuits for years and got by. As you may know, Gore-Tex is great because it breathes. It does an excellent job of keeping water out, yet when your body heats up, you perspire less because air is able to circulate underneath the fabric. Gore-Tex is not perfect, but it is a vast improvement over other fabrics.

You might think that in the summer months you wouldn't need a rainsuit or a jacket. Our experience has shown us otherwise. We have been caught in downpours on the Parkway with no choice but to will away the chill from a body-drenching rain. If nothing else, a rainsuit or jacket will help keep you warm.

In spring and fall, the temperature can fluctuate quite a bit. Chilly temperatures make tights or leg and arm warmers a good idea. A synthetic top is a good item to have on hand, even in the summer, for sudden drops in temperature. You should keep in mind that the mountains can be chilly even at the height of summer. Other than these few specifics, let personal taste dictate your choices.

One common mistake for touring cyclists is to pack too much stuff. You may not need as much clothing as you think. If you do laundry along the way, you should be able to get by with less.

ZIP-TOP BAGS

While we're on the subject of packing gear, we would like to sing the praises of one magic item: zip-top bags. This simple household item is indispensable for keeping your gear dry. Panniers, and other bicycle bags, are not entirely waterproof. In a downpour, zip-top bags will save you from a soggy mess. They also force you to pack more judiciously, since even the gallon-size bags will only hold so much.

HELMETS

It is a grave mistake not to wear a helmet when bicycling. There is no valid reason for not wearing one. We sincerely urge you to wear a helmet at all times while cycling and to wear it properly– not cocked back away from your forehead or unfastened.

LIGHTING SYSTEMS

Due to the frequency of rain, fog, and tunnels on these highways, the National Park Service requires some type of lighting system. Front and rear lights could save your life. Not only do lighting systems make you more visible to cars in inclement weather, but they also help you find your way through the longer tunnels. Some of the tunnels you will encounter are long enough, or curved enough, to leave you in total darkness. Not only can cars inflict injury, but you can easily hurt yourself by taking a spill on a rock or running into the wall of a tunnel.

We use a flashing belt beacon for the rear of our bikes and a white light for the front. Generator- and battery-operated lights each have advantages. Carrying extra bulbs and batteries is a good idea, as some of the smaller bike shops do not stock every type of bulb.

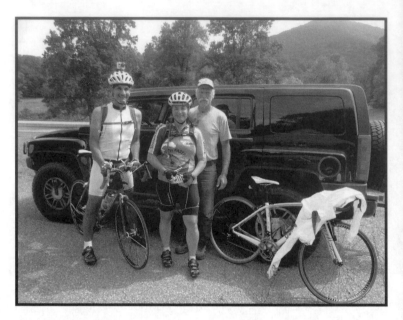

Cyclists meet up with their support-and-gear (SAG) wagon at Peaks of Otter.

GARMIN OR GPS

We first toured the Parkway with a simple bicycle odometer back in the '80s. Now GPS technology enables cyclists to compile data on everything from maps and topography to heart rate and cadence. With a Garmin and a smartphone, you can be very connected to information. However, cell service is very spotty along Skyline Drive and the Parkway. Your phone might as well be useless depending on your service provider at least 50% of the time.

THE CHECKLIST

Finally, we provide you with a master list of the things you should think about taking for the long haul. If you are going out on weekend trips, you can obviously omit some things. We have learned the hard way about carrying too much gear on a bicycle. In 1985 we cycled halfway across the country before we learned how to pack efficiently. To our relief, we finally had it right when we toured Skyline Drive. We cycled from Front Royal to Asheville without a wobble. If you can get by with less, do it.

WHAT TO BRING FOR AN EXTENDED TOUR OF THE BLUE RIDGE

* Cycling shorts, two pairs
* T-shirts or cycling jerseys, two or three
* Thermal underwear (Capilene, CoolMax, or something similar), one
* Running shorts, one pair
* Shorts, one pair
* Gore-Tex rainsuit
* Lightweight wind jacket
* Swimsuit
* Socks, underwear, and so on
* Cycling gloves
* Cycling hat, optional
* Cycling helmet, highly recommended
* Cycling shoes
* Shoes, alternate pair
* Sandals or flip-flops, optional
* Towel, one (as lightweight as you can find)
* Toiletries
* First-aid kit
* Garmin, odometer, or sports watch and charger
* Smartphone and charger
* Sunglasses
* Sunscreen
* Camera and film
* Notepad, pens, stamps, and so on
* Flashlight, small
* Cookstove, fuel, and matches
* Mess kit (don't forget the can opener)
* Rope (a multipurpose item)
* Lightweight sleeping bag and pad
* Tent and ground cloth

Skyline Drive and the Blue Ridge Parkway

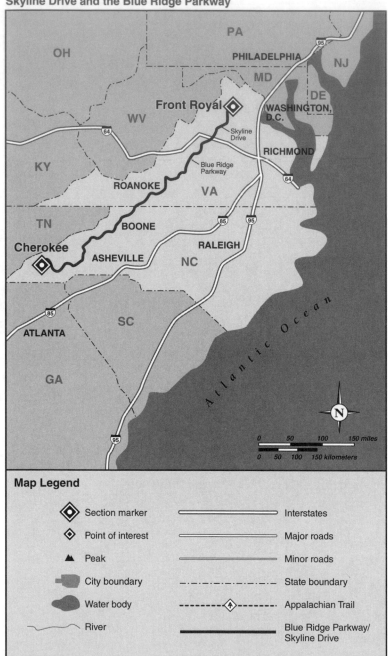

PART 2
Point-by-Point Descriptions

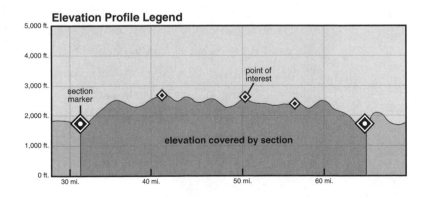

Elevation Profile Legend

An Explanation of Our Point-by-Point Descriptions

In our point-by-point breakdown of Skyline Drive and the Parkway, we list motels, lodges, restaurants, grocery stores, and campgrounds on and off these roads. We also list area hospitals and any bicycle shops within a reasonable distance. Bicycle shops are not in abundance. Because of this, we also list hardware stores that might help you out of a jam.

Our criteria for including facilities off these roads take several factors into account. We have not ventured more than 5 miles off these roads except to visit a few towns we choose to highlight. In most cases, we have not included facilities more than 1–3 miles off the road. We have investigated all side roads except those that are strictly residential. We do not recommend roads that involve extreme descents unless there is something on that road to justify an arduous climb back up.

We have not rated the quality of facilities, although we do make remarks about those that made a favorable impression on us.

We begin at Milepost 0 on Skyline Drive and travel south. If you decide to travel north, just work backward from specific mileposts. Generally, we divide our sections by National Park Service facilities. In some cases, a town will be the dividing point.

There are as many approaches to bicycling in the Blue Ridge as there are riders. A strong rider with gear could reasonably tour Skyline Drive in two days. Unencumbered by gear, one could cycle Skyline Drive in a single day. Then again, there are so many things to see along the way, and so many trails to hike, that spending a week there would not be unreasonable.

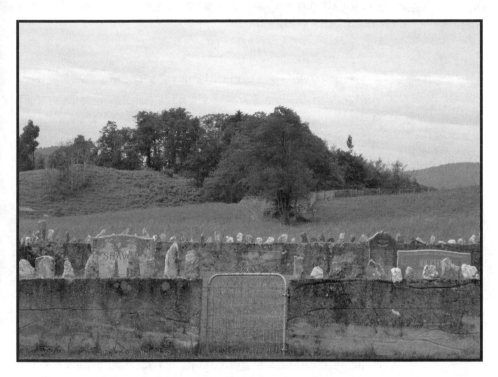

Family graveyard along the Parkway near Roanoke

Special note on Parkway closures: At the time of publication, the National Park Service verified all noted closures of campgrounds and facilities through the 2014 season. The NPS is working to secure concessionaires for privately run facilities (such as Doughton Park and Crabtree Meadows). The NPS is also evaluating closures, and a long-range plan to reopen Parkway facilities in 2015 is forthcoming. As always, please visit **nps.gov/blri** for the latest closures and road conditions.

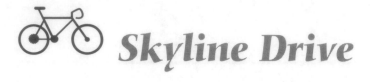

Skyline Drive

Skyline Drive is a scenic highway that runs the length of Shenandoah National Park for a total of 105.5 miles. Shenandoah National Park (hereafter referred to as the Park) is made up of 195,000 acres near George Washington and Jefferson National Forests in western Virginia. Not only does the scenic highway dissect the Park, but 95 miles of the Appalachian Trail are also within park boundaries.

As you cycle along Skyline Drive, the Shenandoah Valley runs parallel to the west, while the Piedmont extends eastward toward the coast. Small details in the construction of Skyline Drive give it a slightly different atmosphere from the Blue Ridge Parkway. Stone and mortar walls grace the edge of the road as it winds along the Blue Ridge Mountains. These structures and the tendency of the trees to form a canopy over the road give Skyline Drive a secluded feeling.

Because Skyline Drive runs continuously through national forest lands, wildlife may be more prevalent here than along the Parkway. A large Virginia white-tailed deer population exists in the Park. You are guaranteed to spot deer at dawn or dusk. Black bears also inhabit the Park. Bear sightings have become more frequent over the years, as evidenced by the bear-proof trash cans and bear poles found at campgrounds and picnic areas. Other wildlife includes red foxes, gray foxes, striped skunks, spotted skunks, bobcats, raccoons, beavers, groundhogs, and chipmunks. About 200 species of birds fly through the Park. Among the larger birds in the Park, you will find wild turkeys, ravens, and ruffed grouse.

Trees in the George Washington National Forest are primarily young second growth as a result of heavy timbering practiced before the Park was established. The primary species include oak and hickory, but you will also find black locust, hemlock, yellow birch, black birch, basswood, tulip poplar, red maple, and sugar maple.

If bicycle touring in the mountains is a new experience for you, Skyline Drive is a good place to start. Facilities abound, with 25 miles being the largest gap between a source of food and the highway. There are two lodges, four restaurants, four camp stores, and four campgrounds in the space of 105 miles. In addition, all but one of the campgrounds have showers. That is pretty good, especially when compared to those along the Parkway. Because this is a national park, there is an entry fee of $5, good for seven consecutive days.

Now that your basic needs have been provided, you are free to concentrate on some very pleasant bicycling. The grades on Skyline Drive are not as severe as those on the Parkway. The longest climbs and descents are at the northern and southern entrances. The elevation drops to 1,390 feet at the Front Royal entrance and 1,900 feet at the Rockfish Gap entrance near Waynesboro.

Skyline Drive: Front Royal to Thornton Gap

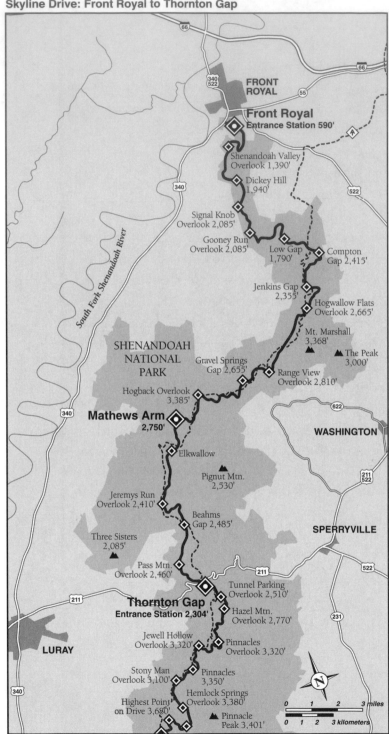

FRONT ROYAL

Front Royal
Entrance Station 590'

Shenandoah Valley
Overlook 1,390'

Dickey Hill
1,940'

Signal Knob
Overlook 2,085'

Gooney Run
Overlook 2,085'

Low Gap
1,790'

Compton
Gap 2,415'

Jenkins Gap
2,355'

Hogwallow Flats
Overlook 2,665'

Mt. Marshall
3,368'

The Peak
3,000'

SHENANDOAH
NATIONAL
PARK

Gravel Springs
Gap 2,655'

Range View
Overlook 2,810'

Hogback Overlook
3,385'

Mathews Arm
2,750'

WASHINGTON

Elkwallow

Pignut Mtn.
2,530'

Jeremys Run
Overlook 2,410'

Beahms
Gap 2,485'

SPERRYVILLE

Three Sisters
2,085'

Pass Mtn.
Overlook 2,460'

Tunnel Parking
Overlook 2,510'

Thornton Gap
Entrance Station 2,304'

Hazel Mtn.
Overlook 2,770'

Jewell Hollow
Overlook 3,320'

Pinnacles
Overlook 3,320'

LURAY

Stony Man
Overlook 3,100'

Pinnacles
3,350'

Hemlock Springs
Overlook 3,380'

Highest Point
on Drive 3,680'

Pinnacle
Peak 3,401'

South Fork Shenandoah River

0   1   2   3 miles

0   1   2   3 kilometers

N

Front Royal to Thornton Gap [0–31.5]

Front Royal, Virginia, is one of the most popular starting points for extended tours of the Blue Ridge. The closest airports to Front Royal are approximately 70 miles away in Washington, D.C. You can cycle out of either Dulles International Airport or Washington National Airport to Front Royal.

When you enter Shenandoah National Park on a bicycle, you experience the sensation of being transported into a separate world. At the height of summer the vegetation is thick and alive with secrets, as if you were traveling through an enchanted forest. The deeper you go, the more entranced you become. Kudzu climbs greedily in the lower elevations. On hot days there is steamy humidity. Slowly, you climb from Front Royal to the higher elevations.

The fact is that you have to do some work to reach the Blue Ridge proper. The first 10 miles of Skyline Drive climb Dickey Ridge before connecting with the Blue Ridge mountain range at Compton Gap (Milepost 10.4). You climb nearly 2,800 feet in this 22-mile stretch up to 3,385 feet at Hogback Overlook.

Numerous overlooks are in this section. At most of these overlooks the Shenandoah River is visible. Take note of the Massanutten Ridge, which divides the Shenandoah Valley for nearly 50 miles. When you study the rock along Skyline Drive, you are looking at molten lava flows called the Catoctin formation.

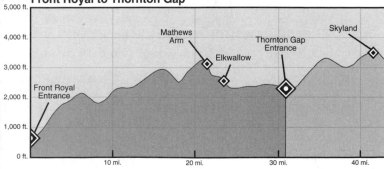

Front Royal to Thornton Gap

Mathews Arm is the first campground on Skyline Drive as you travel south. There is no food here, but Elkwallow Wayside is just 2 miles south with a restaurant and camp store. Three hikes originate from the campground: Traces Trail, Knob Mountain, and Overall Run Falls. From Mathews Arm, you travel another 10 miles, dipping down to 2,304 feet at the Thornton Gap Entrance Station.

MILEPOST

00.0   FRONT ROYAL, VIRGINIA (elevation 590')

Front Royal is situated at the north entrance of Skyline Drive. Facilities include a post office, hospital, numerous restaurants, and motels—but no bicycle shop. The closest pro shop is 18 miles away in Winchester (see Appendix A). All lodging mentioned below is reached by turning right off Skyline Drive and driving north on US 340.

Woodward House on Manor Grade   800-635-7011, 540-635-7010; acountryhome.com $$$
Located at 413 S Royal Ave., three blocks north of Skyline Drive at US 340 and US 55.

Center City Motel   540-635-4050 $

Scottish Inn   540-636-6168 $–$$

Shenandoah Motel   540-635-3181 $
Located 2.5 miles north on US 340 at 1600 N Shenandoah Ave.

4.6   DICKEY RIDGE VISITOR CENTER (elevation 1,940')

The information center has a ranger on duty to answer questions. This facility includes exhibits, a gift shop, water, restrooms, a picnic area, and a nature trail. There is no camping or food here. Open mid–April–August.

21.0   HOGBACK OVERLOOK (elevation 3,385')

This is the highest point so far. Hogback Overlook affords excellent views of the Shenandoah Valley and Shenandoah River.

22.2   MATHEWS ARM (elevation 2,750')   540-999-3132

A steep, 0.8-mile descent leads to the most primitive campground on Skyline Drive; there are no showers or laundry facilities. If you need supplies, the Elkwallow Wayside lies 2 miles south. There are 179 campsites here, each $16 per night, open mid-May–October.

24.1   ELKWALLOW WAYSIDE AND PICNIC AREA

A grill serves breakfast and other simple fare, and there's also a gift shop and a store with groceries and camping supplies. Open April–August. Water and a comfort station are available in the picnic area. The trail to Jeremy's Run, one of the major trout streams in the park, originates here.

31.5   THORNTON GAP (elevation 2,304')
US 211/522

Restrooms and water are available, and you can view Marys Rock from here.

Thornton Gap to Swift Run Gap [31.5–65.5]

The numerous overlooks and hiking trails highlighting streams, waterfalls, and geologic formations are good reasons for taking your time along Skyline Drive. At Thornton Gap you can view Marys Rock, which is formed of granodiorite. Marys Rock Tunnel, just south of Thornton Gap, is the only tunnel on Skyline Drive. As you make your way south toward Skyland Lodge, views of Pinnacles and the profile of Stony Man Mountain dominate the area.

South of Skyland, as you approach the highest point on Skyline Drive (elevation 3,680'), Hawksbill Mountain dominates the skyline as the highest peak in Shenandoah National Park (elevation 4,051'). The Franklin Cliffs Overlook between Mileposts 49 and 50 has great rocky cliffs, perfect for a siesta on a sunny day. If you have time for an hour's hike, Dark Hollow Falls is a good choice at Milepost 50.7, just north of Big Meadows.

The trailhead to Bearfence Mountain summit is found at Milepost 56.4. The hike is a little less than a mile round-trip for a 360-degree view of the area. From this rocky summit you can see Massanutten Ridge and Shenandoah Valley, as well as Grindstone, Green, Powell, and Smith Mountains to the west. To the east, a dozen peaks are within view–Hazeltop, Bush Mountain, Laurel Gap, and Buzzard Rocks among them. This hike is only a mile

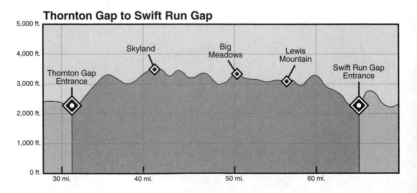

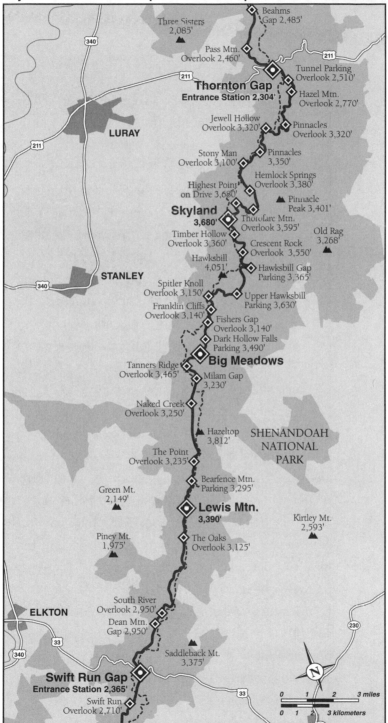

from Lewis Mountain. You might want to drop your gear, set up camp, and cycle back for a hike.

Another reason for taking your time: visiting the park's two lodges–Skyland and Big Meadows. While plenty of camping possibilities are in this section, you may want to consider spending a night at one or both of these lodges. Both are spectacular places to lay your head. If you choose not to spend the night at Skyland, consider having lunch there. The dining room at Skyland is filled with windows ideal for gazing at the Shenandoah Valley. When we think of Big Meadows, the other lodge, two things immediately come to mind: blueberries and deer. Deer sightings are possible at all times of the day. At dawn and dusk, the meadow directly across from the visitor center attracts anywhere from 10 to 50 grazing deer. Take note that the meadow is filled with blueberries ripe for picking in July and August.

Big Meadows is the most extensive facility on Skyline Drive. The campground here uses a reservation system, and reservations are required starting May 14 until it closes at the end of November; call 877-444-6777 up to three months in advance. Big Meadows Lodge has a cozy, rustic charm. We spent two memorable days fogged and rained in here one September. The dining room and great room of the lodge have high ceilings with exposed beams and wrought-iron ceiling fixtures. The massive stone fireplace in the great room has a magnetic force on foul-weather days.

Big Meadows is a major stop for hikers on the Appalachian Trail. The camp store here is superbly stocked. Food items have been selected in sizes and types suitable for campers. The camp store sells clothing, such as parkas and jeans, and supplies, such as candles, Coleman fuel, and toiletries. Big Meadows is the halfway point on Skyline Drive. A strong rider could easily cover

Skyline Drive in two days with Big Meadows being the logical overnight stop.

If you plan on camping at the halfway point on Skyline Drive, Lewis Mountain is a good alternative to Big Meadows. Lewis Mountain Campground has fewer campsites than Big Meadows, but the atmosphere is less hectic, without the constant flow of traffic that the larger complex attracts. A few housekeeping cabins are also available here; they require a reservation.

If you are heading south, you have a great 1,000-foot descent to Swift Run Gap, one of four entrance stations on Skyline Drive.

MILEPOST

32.2 MARYS ROCK TUNNEL (670 feet)
This is the only tunnel in Shenandoah National Park, and one of only two in Virginia.

36.7 PINNACLES
This picnic area is a point of access to the Appalachian Trail. Rustic restrooms and water are available.

41.7 ENTRANCE TO SKYLAND RESORT (elevation 3,680')
Skyland Resort   540-999-2211 $$–$$$
It's a 0.5-mile ride to Skyland's lodge, cabins, restaurant, taproom, and gift shop. There is no camping here. Open April–November.

46.7 UPPER HAWKSBILL PARKING AREA (elevation 3,630')
Hawksbill Mountain (elevation 4,051') is the highest point within park boundaries. The trail to the summit is 2 miles round-trip.

50.7 DARK HOLLOW FALLS (elevation 3,425')
The trail to the falls is 1.5 miles round-trip.

51.0 BIG MEADOWS

Harry F. Byrd, Sr. Visitor Center
Exhibits on history and development of Skyline Drive. While restrooms and water are available year-round, the visitor center is open April–August.

Big Meadows Lodge   540-999-2221 $$–$$$
A 1.1-mile road leads to a rustic lodge, cabins, dining facilities, a taproom, and gift shop. Big Meadows has a campground with showers, laundry facilities, and an excellent camp store. The campground has 217 sites. The visitor center conducts a variety of natural-ist's programs each day. Campground rates are $20 per night; open April–November. For reservations call 877-444-6777 or go to **recreation.gov.**

56.4 BEARFENCE MOUNTAIN PARKING AREA
The hike to the summit is only 0.8 mile round-trip.

57.5 LEWIS MOUNTAIN (elevation 3,390')
540-999-2255, 800-999-4714 $$ (cabins)
You will find complete facilities here, including a campground, housekeeping cabins, showers, laun-dry facilities, and a camp store (open May–August). The camp store has food and camping equipment on half the scale of the Big Meadows store. Lewis Moun-tain has 31 campsites. Rates are $15 per night, and it's open April–October.

62.6 SOUTH RIVER PICNIC AREA

65.5 SWIFT RUN GAP—US 33 (elevation 2,365')
The town of Elkton lies to the west. The elevation differ-ence between the gap and the town is 1,400 feet.

Swift Run Gap to Rockfish Gap [65.5–105.5]

From Swift Run Gap southward, there is a mixed bag of up and down, but the road ultimately climbs into the Loft Mountain area. Loft Mountain Wayside is directly off Skyline Drive. However, the road to the campground is an uphill challenge. If Loft Mountain Campground is your destination for the day, save some energy for the climb to the top.

Loft Mountain Campground has some outstanding campsites. It is worth dragging your bike down into one of the more secluded wooded sites. Deer wander freely through these areas. The Appalachian Trail is no more than 100 yards from one side of the campground; it's great to have just beyond your tent. You can hike a stretch and ponder the differences between experiencing the Blue Ridge by foot and by bicycle.

From Loft Mountain, it is 25 miles to the end of Skyline Drive and the beginning of the Blue Ridge Parkway. If you are heading south, you have an easy descent into Rockfish Gap. If you are heading north toward Loft Mountain, you can expect a steady climb much of the way (nearly a 1,000-foot gain).

For travelers doing a long-distance tour of Skyline Drive and the Parkway, Waynesboro is a good overnight stop. With medical facilities and a full range of shopping opportunities, Waynesboro is one of the few cities in close proximity to Skyline Drive and the Parkway–about 4 miles west of Rockfish Gap. The only disadvantage of a stopover in Waynesboro is that you will start out with a 4-mile climb from the town proper back up to Skyline Drive. Fortunately, if lodging and food are all you require, there are two motels just off Skyline Drive at Rockfish Gap.

Northbounders who need the services of a bike shop should take advantage of the one here; the next accessible bike

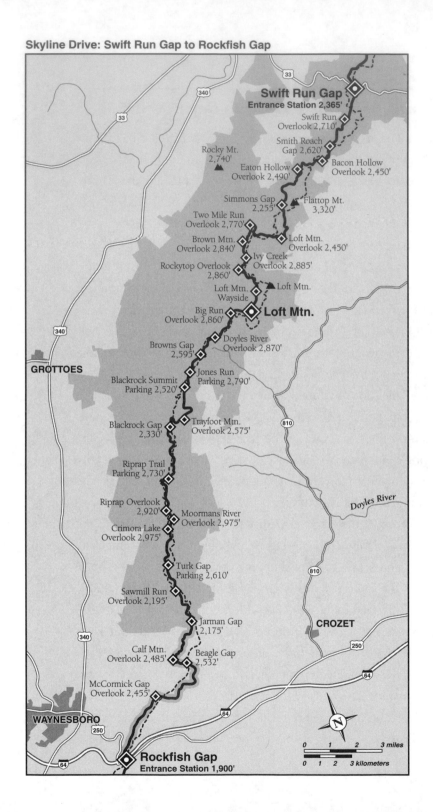

shop is past the end of Skyline Drive in Winchester, about 120 miles away. For southbounders, the next shop is 50 miles away in Lexington.

MILEPOST

79.5   LOFT MOUNTAIN

Loft Mountain Wayside
The wayside has an information area, gift shop, comfort station, water, and grill, which serves breakfast and lunch fare. Open May–October.

Loft Mountain Campground   434-823-4675
There is a steep, 1-mile climb to the campground. The adjoining camp store is well-stocked with camp gear and groceries. Showers and laundry facilities make this a good stop for those doing extended tours. If you're heading south, this is your last chance for shower and laundry facilities in a National Park Service campground. Loft Mountain has almost 200 campsites. Rates are $16 per night; it's open late May–August.

105.4   ROCKFISH GAP—US 250 (elevation 1,909')
Rockfish Gap marks the end of Skyline Drive. After this, the road becomes the Blue Ridge Parkway. Exit here for

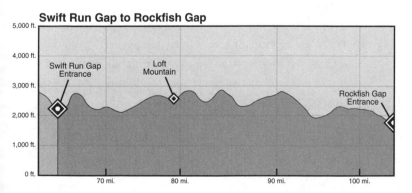

Swift Run Gap to Rockfish Gap

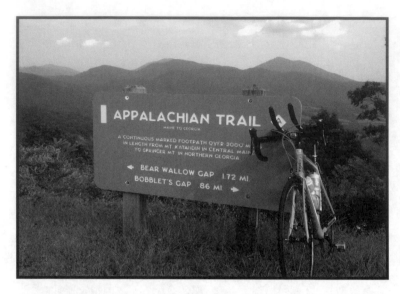

The Appalachian Trail parallels Skyline Drive and intersects the Parkway at several points.

Waynesboro. Take US 250 West 4 miles into Waynesboro, which has a post office, hospital, lodging, restaurants, and a bicycle shop. There are two motels at Rockfish Gap, which should spare a descent into town.

Inn at Afton   540-942-5201 $$

Located on the west side. After exiting the parkway, take an immediate left up VA 601. The inn is on US 250 East.

Colony House Motel   540-942-4156 $–$$

This popular stop for hikers as well as cyclists is located 0.8 mile west on US 250. Continental breakfast is included. It also has a pool and laundry facilities. Local restaurants offer free delivery.

**Rockfish Gap Outfitters   540-943-1461;
rockfishgapoutfitters.com**
This bicycle and outdoors shop is located 3 miles
west on US 250 heading into town at 1461 E Main St.
Hours: Monday–Saturday, 10 a.m.–6 p.m.; Sunday,
noon–5 pmm.

The Blue Ridge Parkway

With little fanfare, the Blue Ridge Parkway begins at Rockfish Gap and continues south for 470 miles. The mile markers still record the terminus of the Parkway at 469 miles even though the construction of the Linn Cove Viaduct added an extra mile. Whereas Skyline Drive is enclosed by national forests, the Parkway winds its way through some disparate geographic situations. The Parkway skirts around two fairly large cities, Roanoke and Asheville. Yet, the Parkway does take you through rugged wilderness areas, such as Shining Rock, Linville Gorge, and Pisgah National Forest. Any single–day trip by bicycle along the Parkway can leave you with distinctly different impressions. One day you roll past cabbage patches and rust-colored barns; the next day your surroundings are craggy, rocky, and downright mountainous.

When you're speeding down the side of a mountain, it's easy to experience sensory overload. Greens blur, the wind roars in your ears, and your adrenaline rises with a rush of feeling. The numerous, inevitable ascents of the Parkway, whether they be 0.25 mile or 6 miles long, are the best times to take note of the flowers, animals, rocks, and trees that surround you.

Once again, trees dominate the natural scene in the Blue Ridge. In his book *A Naturalist's Blue Ridge Parkway*, David Catlin devotes an entire chapter to the integral role trees play. He explains:

> *It is difficult to overstate the importance of trees in the natural history of the mountains, for trees greatly determine not only the kinds, but the character of life here. It can even be legitimately claimed that trees put the 'Blue' in Blue Ridge, for hydrocarbons released into the atmosphere by the forest contribute to the characteristic haze on these mountains and to their distinctive color.*

There are many distinct forests in the Blue Ridge. In the lower elevations there are oak-chestnut, cove hardwood, and

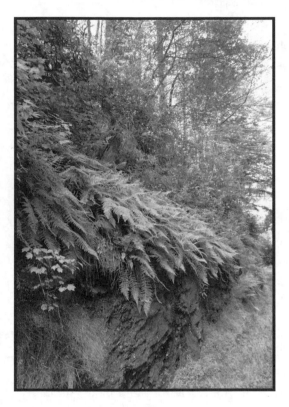

Lush ferns and moss along the roadside in every shade of green

oak-pine forests. The oak–chestnut forests are primarily white, northern red, black, scarlet, and chestnut oaks. The chestnut tree was once prominent along the Blue Ridge, but the chestnut blight fungus wiped out these valuable trees around the turn of the 20th century.

Cove hardwood forests thrive in damp soils. These also feature tulip, sugar maple, yellow buckeye, basswood, beech, yellow birch, northern red oak, and black cherry trees. Areas with good examples of cove hardwood forests include the James River Visitor Center and, closer to the Smokies, Standing Rock Overlook and Big Witch Tunnel.

Oak-pine forests exist in drier, sandier soils, especially around the Asheville area. Species of southern Appalachian pines include white pine, shortleaf pine, pitch pine, Virginia pine, and Table Mountain pine.

In the higher elevations of 5,000 feet or more are northern hardwoods and spruce-fir forests. The northern hardwoods include trees found in the woods of Pennsylvania, New York, and New England. Beech, yellow buckeye, and yellow birch are all found.

The areas with spruce-fir forests are among the most memorable along the Parkway. Found in the very highest elevations, red spruce and Fraser fir are the distinctive inhabitants of Mount Mitchell, Richland Balsam, and Waterrock Knob. Unfortunately, environmental stresses, both man-made and natural, are threatening these trees. The combined effects of acid rain and the woolly aphid have left extensive stands of dying Fraser firs. The bone-white, leafless trunks and limbs are blatant reminders that environmental conditions are poor in the higher elevations.

The grass and heath balds along the Parkway are entirely devoid of trees. In areas such as Craggy Gardens, entire mountainsides are blanketed in rhododendrons and mountain laurels. In May and June, a day of cycling along the Parkway is a study in pinks, from pale to bold.

While we are on the subject of flowers, we would like to tell you when the most notable flowers bloom in the Blue Ridge, so you can be on the lookout.

✳   Dogwood trees show their flowers from mid- to late April.
✳   Spring wildflowers pop up from late March to mid-May.
✳   Flame azaleas display a fantastic orange in May.
✳   Mountain laurels bloom late May–June.
✳   Purple rhododendrons begin sprouting in mid-June.
✳   White rhododendrons show up in June and July.

This schedule applies to Skyline Drive as well. An excellent, detailed bloom calendar of wildflowers along the Parkway can be found in Catlin's book *A Naturalist's Blue Ridge Parkway*. Catlin outlines peak bloom times and mileposts where specific flowers are most likely to be seen.

Much of the Parkway passes through wilderness areas, but scenes of rolling pasture and farmland also border the Parkway for mile upon mile. Roanoke Valley, much of Rocky Knob, Mabry Mill, Doughton Park, Boone, and Blowing Rock consist of farmland. Cabbage and corn are the primary crops grown in these areas. Much of the open hillsides are used for grazing cattle.

Apple trees are common along the Parkway; there is one major orchard right alongside the Parkway between Linville Falls and Little Switzerland. Grapes are also grown in the Blue Ridge. The vineyards of Chateau Morrisette are visible along the mountainside between Rocky Knob and Mabry Mill.

With the Parkway's often narrow boundaries and its proximity to populated areas, you must be very attentive to spot wildlife. Whereas white-tailed deer are commonplace along Skyline Drive, it is unusual to spot them along the Parkway. Deer are very skittish and bound off as soon as you approach them. That's one advantage of traveling by bicycle. You are quiet enough to get within close range of wildlife. Woodchucks and other small mammals often forage alongside the road. Once, we set out on a dusk ride, intent on spotting deer, and nearly wrecked trying to avoid a skunk that had wandered out onto the road. Time spent hiking or camping will reveal cottontail rabbits, raccoons, opossums, and squirrels.

The bird that has fascinated us most along the Parkway is the hawk. Broad-winged and red-tailed hawks are the most common in the Blue Ridge. Often a quick break at an overlook becomes much more when hawks are sighted soaring on the thermal updrafts that carry them for miles.

With all this said about the flora and fauna along the Parkway, there is one thing to remember: elevation is the single overriding factor in bicycling the Parkway. It affects change in natural habitat, terrain, and weather. Elevation influences the road grades of the Parkway, determines the type of forest you cycle past, and is a factor in the weather you encounter. There are journeys within journeys along the Parkway. One day you roll alongside pastures in the 1,000- to 2,000-foot range; another day yields the challenge of 5,000- to 6,000-foot mountains.

While the Parkway does a great job of indicating major intersections and points of interest, it prohibits businesses from advertising directly on the Parkway. While some stores and hotels are easily visible from the Parkway, others are not. Be aware that roadways are marked by unobtrusive brown signs indicating road names and route numbers. Finding the proper roads is particularly challenging between Milepost 136 south and Milepost 380.

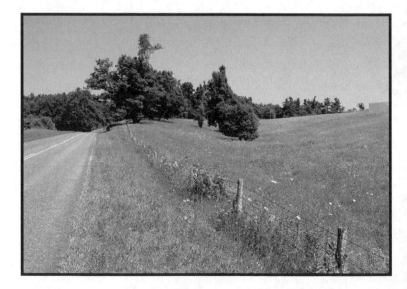

Meadows and farmland are frequent boundaries to the Parkway.

Rockfish Gap to James River Visitor Center
[0.0–64.0]

In the 115 miles from Rockfish Gap to Roanoke, the Blue Ridge narrows to a single ridgetop, which the Parkway traverses, alternating from side to side. This 64-mile stretch leading to the James River Visitor Center begins with some stunning mountain overlooks. From Humpback Rocks Visitor Center, the Parkway winds upward to the rocky vantage point of Raven's Roost. If you are traveling north, this is one of your first views of the Shenandoah Valley. The rock in this area, Catoctin greenstone, has a green tint and is part of the lava flows along Skyline Drive. When we last stood on these rocks, the view was of the sun breaking through swift-moving clouds and mist slinking along the flint-gray ridges.

This section is memorable by bicycle for its wide, arcing switchbacks, which are visible for miles ahead. The countryside varies: you will bike past rocky cliffs; forests of hickory, chestnut oaks, and eastern hemlocks; as well as pastures near the Whetstone Ridge wayside.

VA 664 intersects the Parkway at Milepost 13.7. This road is very steep in both directions. There is one fine facility worth visiting, a private resort called Wintergreen. Although expensive, Wintergreen is open to the public and includes lodging, food, shops, horseback riding, swimming, tennis, and golf.

The road to Sherando Lake is up ahead at Milepost 16.5. Sherando is a beautiful recreation area, but you have to descend the mountain to get there. It is 5.2 miles to the entrance and 2 miles farther to the campground.

All told, the elevation varies quite a bit in this stretch. You reach the highest point north of the James River at 3,334 feet and descend to the James River at 649 feet, the lowest elevation on the

The Blue Ridge Parkway: Rockfish Gap to James Visitor Center

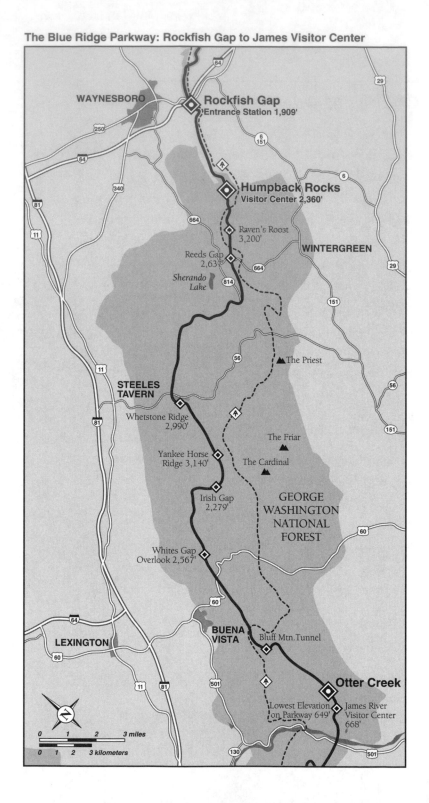

Parkway. This adds up to 4,802 feet climbed from Milepost 0 to Milepost 63. For those traveling north, the climb from the James River brings the total up to 5,990 feet.

If you are planning to make this stretch in one day, Whetstone Ridge may be a welcome break point for travelers in either direction. You will cross the James River just a few miles south of Otter Creek Campground. The James River Visitor Center features a museum and a self-guided walking trail through the river locks system that was designed to accommodate horse-pulled barges through the Blue Ridge. The original plan, developed by George Washington, was to connect waterways that extended into Ohio. Ultimately, railways replaced the barges for transporting goods.

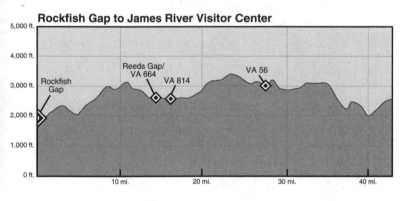

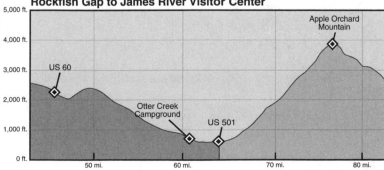

MILEPOST

0.0   ROCKFISH GAP—US 250/I-65 (elevation 1,909')

5.8   HUMPBACK ROCKS VISITOR CENTER (elevation 2,360')
You may want to tour the working farm here. The facilities include water and restrooms. A ranger is on duty.

8.5   HUMPBACK PICNIC AREA
Tables and water

10.7 RAVEN'S ROOST (elevation 3,200')
Take time to perch on these rocks and view the Shenandoah Valley.

13.7 REEDS GAP—VA 664 (elevation 2,637')
Cabin Creekwood   540-943-8552; cabincreekwood.com $$–$$$
Pleasant cabins located on the west side of the Parkway. Steep 1.8-mile descent but closer than Sherando.

Wintergreen   855-699-1858; wintergreenresort.com $$$
Wintergreen is open year-round. Proceed 1 mile east on VA 664. Facilities include lodging, food, gift shops, and recreational facilities.

16.0 VA 814
Royal Oak Country Store and Cabins   540-943-7625; vacabins.com $$$
Located 0.3 mile west off the Parkway, the store has some food supplies and a small deli.

Sherando Lake   540-942-5965
This national forest campground is beautiful, but it is a significant detour off the Parkway proper on VA 814, involving a total of 7.2 miles one-way. Entrance into the park is $1 for bicyclists. The camping fee is

$15–$20 per campsite (open April–October). You will find free hot showers at the bathhouse. A small camp store with limited hours sells basic food items.

27.2   VA 56 (elevation 2,969')

Although this highway is winding, narrow, and steep in either direction, there is one campground 3 miles east of the Parkway.

Montebello Resort   540-377-2650; montebellova.com $–$$$ (cabins)

The campground ($18 per night) and adjacent store are a very steep 3 miles east of the Parkway. The store has snacks and limited groceries. Cabins are also available. Open April–October.

Steeles Tavern Manor   800-743-8666, 540-377-9494; steelestavern.com $$$

Ready for some pampering? It is worth the trek 5.5 miles west of the Parkway, to the town of Steeles Tavern, to stay at this B&B, which offers luxury accommodations and fine dining. There's also an extensive book and video library and a DVD player in each room.

29.0   WHETSTONE RIDGE (elevation 2,990')

This picnic area has water and restrooms. Open May–October.

45.6   US 60 (elevation 2,312')

Lexington Bike Shop   540-463-7969

Need the services of a bike mechanic? It's about 11 miles (3 of them steep) west to the charming town of Lexington and the shop at 130 S Main St. Hours: Monday–Friday, 9 a.m.–noon and 1–5 p.m.; Saturday, 9 a.m.–noon.

53.1   BLUFF MOUNTAIN TUNNEL (630 feet)

This is the first of many tunnels on the Parkway heading south. It is the only one on the Parkway in Virginia.

60.8   OTTER CREEK CAMPGROUND & RESTAURANT

(elevation 777') [closed for 2014]

This is a strategically placed campground for touring cyclists. We hope this campground will reopen in 2015. The campground has 45 tent sites and 24 trailer sites.

63.6   JAMES RIVER VISITOR CENTER (elevation 668') [closed for 2014]

Make sure that you take the time out for the exhibits and the self-guided nature trail to the river locks if the center is open.

63.9   US 501

H & H Food Market & Restaurant   434-299-5153

Follow rolling hills 1 mile east toward Big Island to reach this well-stocked grocery store and adjacent restaurant.

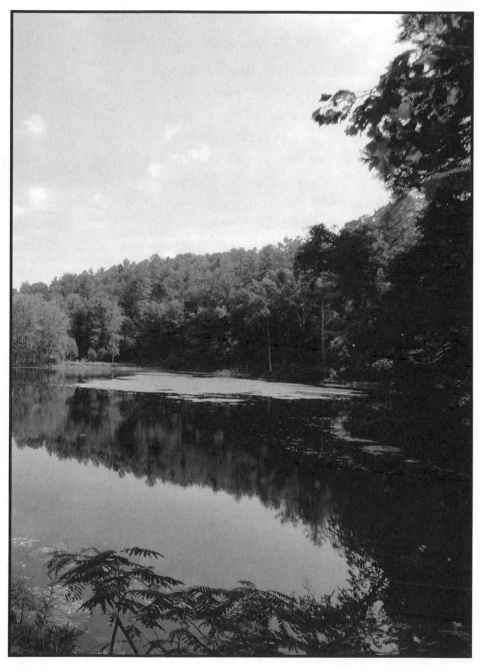

Otter Creek

James River Visitor Center
to Roanoke Mountain [64–121]

Since you are starting out at the lowest point on the Parkway and heading toward the highest point on the Parkway in Virginia, expect to do some climbing. Uphill climbs will amount to 4,000 feet. That's quite a bit for a mere 25 miles.

Midway into your ascent, you will encounter Thunder Ridge at 3,845 feet. This is a thickly forested area of northern red oaks and Carolina hemlocks. From here you will cycle past stands of striped and mountain maples at the overlook of Arnold's Valley. The Appalachian Trail parallels the Parkway throughout this section and crosses it once at Milepost 74.9.

Certainly one reason for the popularity of Peaks of Otter, named for the headwaters of the Otter River, is its proximity to numerous hiking trails. It is also one of the most extensive facilities on the Parkway with a large campground and a modest camp store. The camp store stocks basic food supplies, beverages, and camping supplies. The lodge and restaurant have a simple mountain elegance, from the gray-stained exterior to the high ceilings and exposed beams of the dining room. Views of Sharp Top, Flat Top Mountain, and Abbott Lake provide the crowning touch.

It is 35 miles from Peaks of Otter to Roanoke Mountain. The city of Roanoke sits in a valley, so the majority of this section is downhill. With both an airport and bus service, this city is a possible beginning or ending point for a tour of the Blue Ridge. If you are on an extended tour, it is also the place to seek assistance for any major difficulties. The population of the Roanoke metropolitan area is more than 300,000; Roanoke and Asheville are the largest cities directly off the Parkway.

There are numerous access roads from the Parkway into the Roanoke area. We have investigated each side road in order to

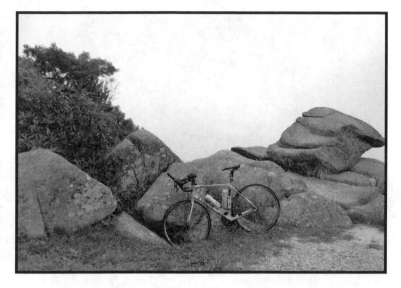

Thunder Ridge Overlook near the highest elevation in Virginia, 3,950 feet

recommend the best ways to safely travel by bike into the city. The Roanoke area provides a key opportunity to stock up on food and supplies. For those seeking motels, there are several possibilities. We discovered an excellent bicycle route into downtown Roanoke (described on page 70), which boasts a farmers market, museums, shops, and restaurants.

The best selection of motels directly off the Parkway is 1.5 miles down US 220 North. Be careful, though: US 220 is a major highway with heavy truck traffic. Fortunately, you can pick up a frontage road, which is just a mile north and is a direct route to most facilities.

The most accessible bicycle shop in the Roanoke area is best reached from the Vinton/US 24 exit (Milepost 112.2).

For anyone considering flying in or out of Roanoke, you should be forewarned that the airport is on the extreme north end of the city. We do not have a route to recommend from the

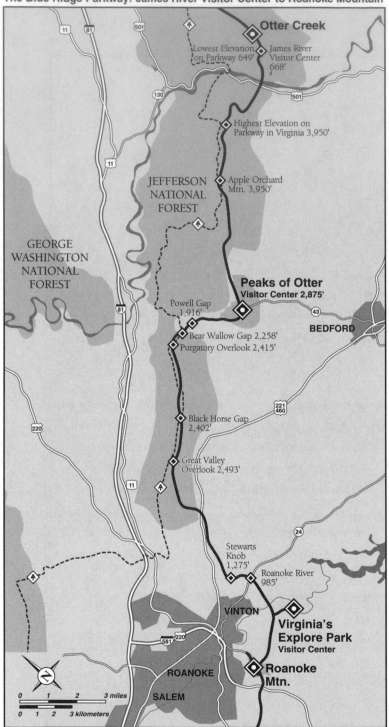

airport to the Parkway. The most direct route is US 220. If you
know you will be cycling from the airport to the Parkway, we
suggest that you get a city map from the Roanoke Valley Convention and Visitors Bureau (see Appendix B).

The Parkway assumes a different character in the Roanoke
area. In the Roanoke Valley, mountains are replaced by rolling
farmland and the presence of a major city. Residential areas are visible from the Parkway. A true-blue naturalist might scoff at the
Roanoke area, yet the opportunity to bicycle in the Blue Ridge at all
is a compromise between people and their technology, and nature.

For an appreciation of the city, we recommend taking in the
view from the overlook at Mill Mountain Park, just a mile from
Roanoke Mountain Campground. A pleasant nature trail at Milepost 115 (Roanoke River Overlook) identifies native trees,

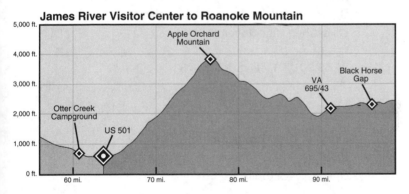

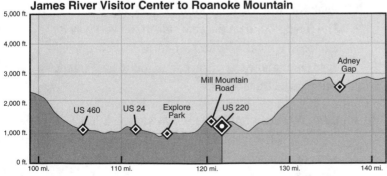

including chestnut oak, eastern hemlock, black locust, sassafras, scarlet oak, and white pine. The trail culminates in an overlook of the Roanoke River.

For those traveling north to Peaks of Otter, the going is uphill. Since you are climbing up out of the Roanoke Valley, you will gain a total of 2,608 feet. Make sure to save some energy for the last 5 miles into Peaks of Otter, a tough stretch of steep road.

MILEPOST

76.7 **APPLE ORCHARD MOUNTAIN** (elevation 3,950')
Highest point along Parkway in Virginia

85.6 **PEAKS OF OTTER LODGE** (elevation 2,525')
866-387-9905; peaksofotter.com $$–$$$
Peaks of Otter Lodge was renovated and reopened in 2013. Facilities here include a restaurant, bar, gift shop, and visitor center. Nature trail around Abbott Lake. Open May–November.

85.9 **VA 43 SOUTH** (elevation 2,875')
Take the exit on the east side to head toward Bedford, Virginia.

Peaks of Otter Visitor Center
Small museum, gift store, restrooms, and water. Open May–October.

Peaks of Otter Campground   540-586-1614
The campground on the east side of the Parkway is equipped with a camp store for grocery items, beverages, and sandwiches. The campground has 90 tent sites and 53 trailer sites.

91.0 **BEAR WALLOW GAP—VA 695/VA 43** (elevation 2,258')
The ride to the town of Buchanan is a very steep, 4-mile descent. Not recommended.

97.7   BLACK HORSE GAP (elevation 2,402')

105.8   US 460
A large chain grocery store is located 1 mile west on this very busy highway.

112.2   US 24
Vinton, Virginia
Vinton is a good place to stock up on groceries. Take US 24 west 0.8 mile toward Roanoke to the East Vinton Plaza. US 24 is a four-lane highway with a small shoulder. The East Vinton Plaza has a grocery store, bank, and laundry.

Cardinal Bicycle   540-344-2453; cardinalbicycle.com
From the Vinton exit, follow US 24 west for 1.8 miles. US 24 will turn left, but you should continue straight on Washington Avenue. (It becomes Gus Nicks Boulevard.) At 3.6 miles turn right onto Orange Avenue and proceed 0.5 mile to Cardinal Bicycle on the right. Hours: Monday–Friday, 10 a.m.–7 p.m.; Saturday, 9 a.m.–5 p.m.

Days Inn   540-342-4551 $$
Turn left onto Orange Avenue and go 1.4 miles. Located on left. This road is a major artery and has heavy traffic.

112.9   ROANOKE RIVER OVERLOOK (elevation 985')
It's a 20-minute walk on the Roanoke River Trail to an overlook of the river.

115.0   EXPLORE PARK 540-427-1800; roanokecountyva.gov /index.aspx?NID=1468
Located an easy, rolling 1.5 miles off the Parkway, the park features authentic and reconstructed buildings demonstrating American Indian traditions, colonial frontier culture, and 19th-century life. Nine miles of

mountain bike trails, hiking, fishing, and picnicking
are featured in this 1,100-acre park. Admission
required. Open April–October, Wednesday–Sunday.

120.4   MILL MOUNTAIN ROAD

Mill Mountain Road is the best route to downtown
Roanoke. Ultimately, the road becomes a marked bicycle
route as it parallels the Roanoke River. There is one thing
we want to caution you about: this route is all downhill
going into the city and all uphill going back to the
Parkway. Now is the time to have an enlightened attitude
about climbing hills.

To access downtown Roanoke from the Parkway, turn
onto Mill Mountain Road at Milepost 120.5 on the
Parkway. Follow Mill Mountain Road up, around, and
down the mountain. First you will pass Roanoke Mountain
Campground on the left at 1.2 miles; Mill Mountain Park
is 1.2 miles beyond the campground at 2.4 miles. Then you
will descend down the mountain into Roanoke. Mill
Mountain Road becomes Walnut Street. At 4.4 miles turn
left onto Belleview Avenue. Belleview cuts through the
middle of the Roanoke Memorial Hospital complex at 5
miles, and soon you will see bike-route signs. Belleview
bears right onto Wiley Drive. Wiley Drive meanders alongside the Roanoke River, passes through Smith Park, and
passes twice over the Roanoke River. At the second bridge
take the next left over the railroad crossing onto Winoa
Street. The next street is Main Street. Turn left.

Roanoke Mountain Campground 540-982-9242
[closed for 2014]
Roanoke Mountain Campground is 1.2 miles off the
Parkway on Mill Mountain Road. The only facilities
here are restrooms. A ranger is on duty. The campground has 74 tent sites and 31 trailer sites.

Mill Mountain Zoo (elevation 1,747')   540-343-3241;
mmzoo.org
Mill Mountain Park is located 2.4 miles from the Parkway. It features a zoological park, a wildflower garden,
and an overlook with an outstanding view of Roanoke
and the Roanoke Valley. The park has a snack bar and
restrooms. April–November: daily, 10 a.m.–4:30 p.m.
December–March: Thursday–Sunday, 10 a.m.–
4:30 p.m. Closed December 25. Admission is $7.50 for
ages 12 and up, $5 for ages 3–11.

121.2 US 220 SOUTH

Apple Valley Motel   540-989-0675 $
Located 0.3 mile east of the Parkway on US 220 (5063
Franklin Rd.). Walmart is just across the highway.

121.4 US 220 NORTH

US 220 North is a major highway with heavy truck traffic. Proceed with caution. It is 1.4 miles to a frontage road
that will take you to numerous motels and restaurants
including Starbucks, Fleet Feet Sports, and a large home-
improvement store.

Colony House Motor Lodge   540-345-0411;
colonyhousemotorlodge.com $$
Located 1.5 miles west from the Parkway on US 220
(3560 Franklin Rd.).

East Coasters Bike Shop   540-774-7933;
eastcoasters.com
East Coasters is located about 2 miles from the Park-
way in the Old Country Plaza near Tanglewood Mall.
Call for directions. Open Monday–Friday, 11 a.m.–
7 p.m.; Saturday, 10 a.m.–5 p.m.; Sunday, noon–4 p.m.

Roanoke Mountain to Mabry Mill [121–176]

One of the best things about the climb south, out of Roanoke, is that you have plenty of time to appreciate the views of Roanoke Valley. Between Mileposts 128 and 133, the Parkway climbs 1,800 feet with a 6.8% grade. Your breakfast will be long gone by the time you reach Smart View at Milepost 154.5. You can tell little about road grades along this stretch from studying the Parkway map. It is not safe to assume that, since Rocky Knob is at 3,572 feet and Roanoke is at 1,425 feet, you will have smooth sailing traveling north into Roanoke. Although the map leads you to expect a drop in elevation of 2,147 feet, the Parkway actually rises and descends numerous times. Likewise, these climbs make for welcome descents.

Overall, there are two significant inclines for southbound- ers between Roanoke and Rocky Knob. The first substantial climb begins about 6 miles out of Roanoke. The second major uphill starts around Rakes Millpond at Milepost 162.4 and ends beyond the Rocky Knob Campground at about Milepost 169.

There is one area on this stretch convenient for food and shelter: VA 8 at Tuggle Gap. There you will find good places to stock up on supplies or have breakfast or lunch.

We want to stress the beauty of the Rocky Knob area. Its grassy knobs are similar to those of Scotland. The huge, protrud- ing boulders and rocks are a farmer's nightmare, but the pastoral setting of Rocky Knob is a great place to set up an easel and canvas, or to simply stand and feel the energy of the wind.

The 9 miles between Rocky Knob and Mabry Mill move through the high knobs of the Rocky Knob area, and then swing down to Mabry Mill in one memorable swoop. If you are traveling south and camping at Rocky Knob, we suggest that you break camp early and cycle the vigorous 9 miles to Mabry Mill for buckwheat pancakes. Arrive at Mabry Mill early to avoid standing in line.

If you are traveling north, the climbs into Rocky Knob are rewarding. The most memorable climb of this section reveals itself as a wide, rising arc in full view of the climber.

The big surprise of this section is Chateau Morrisette. Who would be expecting a winery in these parts? Less than a mile off the Parkway at Milepost 171, this is the only winery that we know that is in such close proximity to the Parkway. Take some time out for a tour of the winery and, by all means, the wine tasting.

Mabry Mill is a certified scenic spot on the Parkway. Reported to be the most photographed sight on the Parkway, it is nearly always crowded. Beware of traffic when approaching the area. Mabry Mill is popular for good reason—a tour of the mill is fascinating. They still grind and sell cornmeal and buckwheat flour. Also on exhibit are a moonshine still, a sorghum mill, and a soap-making kettle. On a summer day, you may even chance upon a musician or two playing the hammered dulcimer, banjo, or mandolin.

MILEPOST

135.9   ADNEY GAP (elevation 2,690')
     US 221 has no facilities.

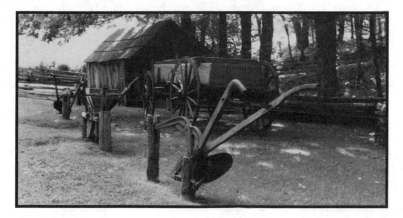

A unique display of antique farming equipment at Mabry Mill

The Blue Ridge Parkway: Roanoke Mountain to Mabry Mill

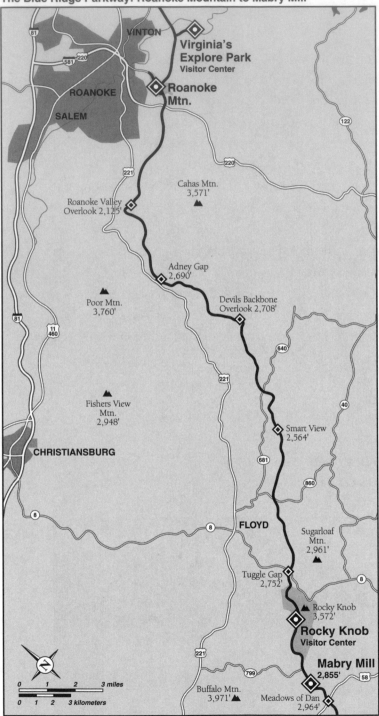

81

VINTON

220

581

220

Virginia's
Explore Park
Visitor Center

ROANOKE

Roanoke
Mtn.

SALEM

122

221

Cahas Mtn.
3,571'

220

Roanoke Valley
Overlook 2,125'

81

Adney Gap
2,690'

Devils Backbone
Overlook 2,708'

11
460

Poor Mtn.
3,760'

640

221

Fishers View
Mtn.
2,948'

40

Smart View
2,564'

CHRISTIANSBURG

681

860

8

8

FLOYD

Sugarloaf
Mtn.
2,961'

8

Tuggle Gap
2,752'

Rocky Knob
3,572'

Rocky Knob
Visitor Center

221

Mabry Mill
2,855'

58

0   1   2   3 miles

0   1   2   3 kilometers

799

Buffalo Mtn.
3,971'

Meadows of Dan
2,964'

Bent Mountain Lodge Bed and Breakfast   540-651-2500; bentmountainlodgebedandbreakfast.com $$-$$$
Exit the Parkway south on US 221 toward Floyd and go 3 miles; turn left just before Copper Hill. Make a left onto Route 647 (Deer Run Road), turn left on Parkway Drive, and turn left on Mountain View Drive. Go to top of Mountain View. Suites and cabins with continental breakfast are great for a side trip to the town of Floyd.

150.9   VA 881/VA 640
Floyd-Franklin Turnpike is to the west and Five Mile Mountain Road is to the east.

154.1   SMART VIEW (elevation 2,564') [closed for 2014]
Smart View is a lovely picnic area with lots of shade for a hot summer day. Restrooms and water are available here. The 2.5-mile Smart View Trail is here.

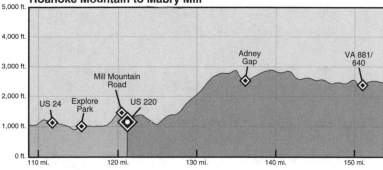

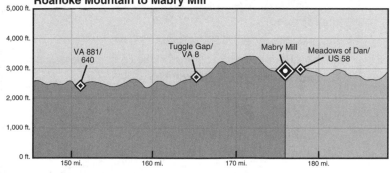

159.5   STONEWALL BED & BREAKFAST   540-745-2861;
stonewallbed.com $$–$$$
Quaint place to rest your head just off the Parkway.
Large country breakfast provided to guests. Special
spaghetti dinners for cyclists on request. Turn onto VA
680 (Shooting Creek Road) on east side of the Parkway; then make an immediate left on Wendi Pate Trail.

165.3   TUGGLE GAP—VA 8 (elevation 2,752')

Tuggles Gap Restaurant & Motel   540-745-3402;
tugglesgap.biz $
Exit onto VA 8 and turn left. Proceed 150 yards. This
place doesn't look like much; the motel is very small,
but the restaurant serves good food.

167.1   ROCKY KNOB CAMPGROUND (elevation 3,572')
540-593-3503
Rocky Knob is among our favorite Parkway campgrounds. You will find an excellent trail system here.
A short but steep walk to the top of Rocky Knob
affords an excellent view. (Watch out for cow pat-
ties.) The campground has 81 tent sites and 28 trailer
sites. Access to the 10.8-mile Rock Castle Gorge Trail.

169.0   ROCKY KNOB VISITOR CENTER   [closed for 2014]
Information center, picnic area, restrooms, phone, and
access to top 3.1-mile Black Ridge Trail.

171.0   CHATEAU MORRISETTE WINERY   276-593-2865;
thedogs.com
Just past Milepost 171, look for VA 726, where you
will turn right if traveling south. Make an immediate
left onto VA 777 (Winery Road). The winery is less
than 0.25 mile from here and is open for tours Monday–
Thursday, 10 a.m.–5 p.m.; Friday–Saturday, 10 a.m.–
6 p.m.; and Sunday, 11 a.m.–5 p.m. Lunch is served
daily; dinner is also served on weekends.

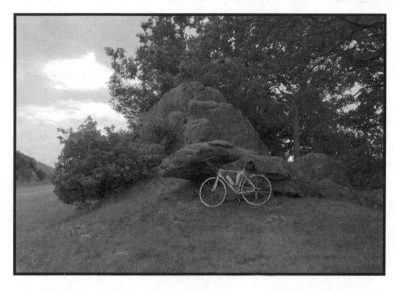

Piles of boulders approaching Rocky Knob

174.0   WOODBERRY INN   540-593-2567; woodberryinn.com
200 yards from the Parkway with a continental
breakfast, restaurant serving dinner, and bar. Turn at
Rocky Knob Cabin sign. Open February–December.

174.1   ROCKY KNOB CABINS   [closed for 2014]

176.2   MABRY MILL (elevation 2,855')   **276-952-2947;
mabrymillrestaurant.com**
Mabry Mill is open May–October. In addition to the
mill and exhibits, there is a gift shop, restaurant,
restrooms, drinking water, and a phone. Restaurant
hours: daily, 8 a.m.–6 p.m.

Mabry Mill to Cumberland Knob [176–217]

The town of Meadows of Dan is just 1 mile south of Mabry Mill. Here you will find ample facilities: groceries, a laundry, restaurants, and lodging.

Relative to other sections, this 23-mile stretch is not very demanding. There is one notable climb, a little over a mile long, as you approach Groundhog Mountain, which rises to an elevation of 3,030 feet. You might want to take a break here, climb to the top of the observation tower, and study the various types of fences on display: snake rail, buck and rail, and post and rail.

From Groundhog Mountain, the road rolls out toward Fancy Gap with no big surprises. The Parkway drops slightly, and you will find a straightaway of considerable length through the Orchard Gap area. Orchard Gap Deli is visible to the left.

We have two great sensory impressions of this area. One is the pungent aroma from the many fields of cabbages ready for harvest in September; the other is an abundance of flame azaleas, which bloom bright orange in May.

There is a slight climb into Fancy Gap, where the elevation is 2,925 feet. Fancy Gap, visible to either side of the Parkway, is an obvious stopping place for those camping or needing a motel. For some, the distance between the National Park Service campgrounds of Rocky Knob and Doughton Park will be farther than you want to push in one day. It all depends on pace and where you are in your trip. Before you pass up the facilities at Fancy Gap, keep in mind that the distance to Doughton Park includes roughly 9 miles of steady climbing, and that the park may be closed.

You will cross from Virginia into North Carolina along this section. As you pedal along a shady, winding stretch of road, the Parkway makes a seamless transition from one state to the other. Upon leaving Fancy Gap, you will encounter a fairly steep climb

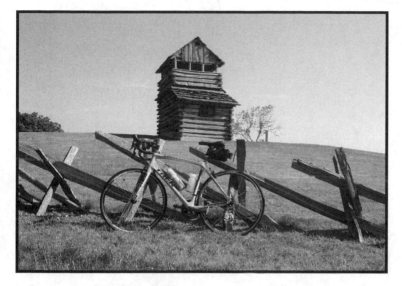

Groundhog Mountain observation tower

of about a mile. There is an equal proportion of up and down all the way to Cumberland Knob.

We made up the term *rolling mountain* while cycling this section. When you look at the road, you just know you'll be cycling rolling hills, the kind that leave you enough momentum to crest the hill ahead of you, but this is rarely the case. Instead, you end up shifting down in the face of a climb, whether it is short or long.

This section of the Parkway is mostly pasture and farmland spread out across rolling hills. Cattle graze on small knobs with farmhouses frequently within view. Small streams trickle haphazardly alongside the Parkway. There's a timeless, down-home feel to this landscape.

Cumberland Knob was the first park constructed on the Parkway. It makes a good break point, or starting point if you are day-tripping.

One big surprise in this section is the presence of an American Youth Hostel. There is no other hostel along Skyline Drive or

The Blue Ridge Parkway: Mabry Mill to Cumberland Knob

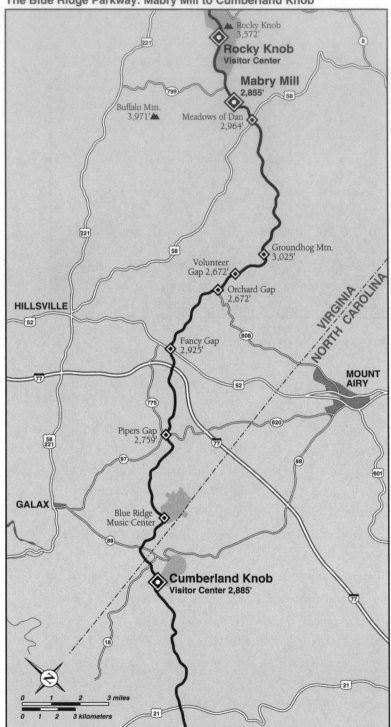

the Parkway. Unless you are a member of AYH, you probably would not know this is here. It is secluded on a wonderful piece of property just off the Parkway. The house is charming, with all the comforts of home, including a great deck in the back.

MILEPOST

177.7   MEADOWS OF DAN—US 58 (elevation 2,964')

Meadows of Dan is visible to either side of the Parkway. The motel and campground are just west of the Parkway; the grocery and restaurant are just east on US 58.

Meadows of Dan Food Market
This full-service grocery is open year-round.

Poor Farmer's Market
This is typical of a country store. You'll find mostly trinkets and souvenirs but also food associated with the country-fresh produce, ham, and locally ground grits and flour.

Mountain House Restaurant   276-952-2999
Typical Southern-style fare, offering breakfast, lunch, and dinner. Open year-round.

Blue Ridge Motel & Restaurant   276-952-2244 $
This motel and restaurant is located 75 yards west on US 58.

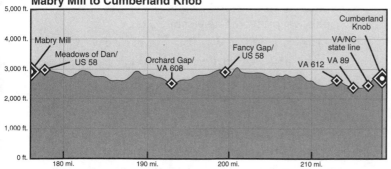

Mabry Mill to Cumberland Knob

**Meadows of Dan Campground   276-952-2292;
meadowsofdancampground.com**
Open year-round with easy access from the Parkway;
go west on US 58 about 0.5 mile. Tent sites are $15;
log cabins are also available.

179.4   ROUND MOUNTAIN VIADUCT

180.5   MAYBERRY TRADING POST
On your left when you're traveling south, this general
store is well-stocked with groceries and baked
goods. On occasion, we have enjoyed traditional
bluegrass music here.

188.8   GROUNDHOG MOUNTAIN (elevation 3,025')
Groundhog Mountain has an observation tower and
features a display of the various types of fences constructed along the Parkway. You will find a picnic area,
restrooms, and drinking water.

189.0   DOE RUN LODGE AND RESTAURANT (elevation 2,950')
276-398-4099; doerunlodging.com $$$
Just visible on the Parkway's east side, Doe Run fea-
tures suites and villas with daily and weekly rates.
Facilities include tennis courts, a pool, and restaurant.

189.9   PUCKETT CABIN PARKING AREA

193.5   ORCHARD GAP—VA 608 (elevation 2,672')
**Volunteer Gap Inn and Cabins   276-398-4323;
aparkwaypieceofheaven.com $$$**
Visible from the Parkway. Take gravel road west
toward large sign. Luxury rooms and cabins; open
year-round.

193.5   RAP'S BAR & GRILL (elevation 2,675')
276-398-2204; rapsva.com
Catering to motorcyclists, Rap's has sandwiches, salads, entrées, basic snacks, and groceries. Live music

on weekends. Open year-round. Hours: daily,
9 a.m.-6 p.m.

Lonesome Pine Cabins   276-398-3332, 888-799-9214;
lonesomepinecabins.net $$
One- and two-story cabins with kitchenettes and
dining areas.

194.7   **THE INN AND COTTAGES AT ORCHARD GAP**
276-398-3206; innatorchardgap.com $$$
Look for Thunder Ridge Road on the west side, go
about 0.2 mile, and turn left on Lightning Ridge Road.

199.4   **FANCY GAP—US 52** (elevation 2,925')
Fancy Gap is visible to either side of the Parkway. Motels,
restaurants, a campground, and a post office are all here.

Mountain Top Restaurant & Motel   276-728-9414   **$**
The restaurant is just east of the Parkway on US 52;
the motel is on the west side. Open year-round.

Lake View Motel & Restaurant   276-728-7841   **$**
Located west on US 52. Open year-round.

Fancy Gap/Blue Ridge Parkway KOA   276-728-7776
Go 0.2 mile west on VA 683. You will see signs for
camping. This excellent campground is open year-
round. Facilities include showers, laundry, camp
store, ice, and telephone.

202.8   **GRANITE QUARRY OVERLOOK** (elevation 3,015')
Good views south of Pilot Mountain State Park and
Hanging Rock

206.5   **FELTS BROTHERS GROCERY**
Just 0.5 mile off the Parkway; heading south on the
Parkway turn right onto VA 608, and then turn left on
VA 97 North. Hours: Monday–Friday, 6 a.m.–8 p.m.;
Saturday, 8 a.m.–6 p.m. It's about 0.5-mile moderate climb
back to the Parkway.

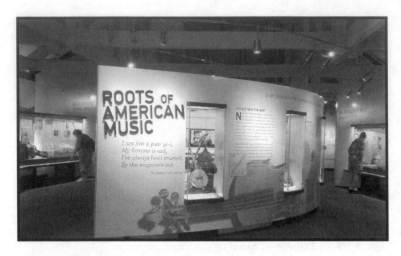

Exhibit at Blue Ridge Mountain Music Center

213.3   VA 612

**Blue Ridge Music Center   276-236-5309;
blueridgemusiccenter.org**
Supported by the National Council for the Traditional
Arts, this venue offers performances by local and
nationally known bluegrass and country musicians.
Open to the public for performances only.

215.8   VA 89

Bits and Pieces Grocery
Open year-round, this store offers snacks and drinks.
If you need more substantial supplies, ride west 5
miles into Galax to Lowe's, a chain grocery store.

216.9   VIRGINIA–NORTH CAROLINA STATE LINE

217.5   CUMBERLAND KNOB (elevation 2,885')

There is no camping or food here. You will find restrooms, drinking water, and a picnic area. A ranger is on
duty at the small gift shop. A brief trail system features a
hike along Gully Creek with views of the Piedmont.

Cumberland Knob to Northwest Trading Post
[217–259]

From Cumberland Knob southward you will encounter rolling hills with panoramic views of the Piedmont to the east. Pastureland, meadows, and apple orchards comprise much of the scenery between Milepost 217 and 230. Milepost 221.5 to Milepost 230.1 is relatively flat. This is one of the rare straightaways on the Parkway where cycling is a breeze–enjoy. Big Pine Creek meanders from one side of the Parkway to the other.

Little Glade Pond (Milepost 230.1) marks a change in terrain. This is a pleasant break point before heading out for the climb into Doughton Park. Conversely, it makes a great place to regroup after tearing down out of the mountains from Doughton Park.

From Little Glade Pond (elevation 2,709'), the Parkway begins a steady 1,000-foot climb, which crests at Air Bellows Gap (elevation 3,729'). The terrain undergoes a subtle metamorphosis from farmland to mountain as you approach the Doughton Park area. Instead of grassy meadows, you begin to cycle past sheer rock face. Doughton Park is one of the larger parks in land area. Although you're only in the 3,000- to 4,000-foot range, south of the lodge the road will thrill you as it cuts right through mountain; you shoot past a high rock wall where the mountain was blasted to make way for the road.

Beware of gaps throughout this entire area, where gusting winds may be encountered. Cycling through gaps at high speeds can be tricky.

Signs announce Doughton Park well before facilities are encountered. Heading south, Brinegar Cabin (Milepost 238.5) is the first point of interest. The campground is next at Milepost 239.2. Deer sightings are a daily occurrence at Doughton Park, especially at dawn and dusk; try the meadow north of the campground.

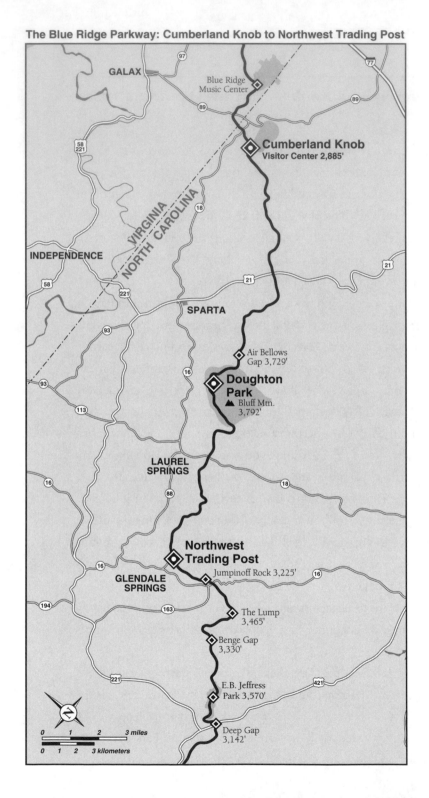

If you stay overnight at Doughton Park, a climb to Bluff Mountain Overlook on the trail system should give you a fine appreciation of the feat you are accomplishing by cycling the Parkway. South from the rocky ledge of Bluff Mountain, the highway twists uphill through decidedly mountainous terrain. In fact, cycling from either direction into Doughton Park is a challenge.

Past the lodge and restaurant at Doughton Park, there are several miles of spectacular mountain scenery and cycling territory. One of the big thrills for us is the view you have of the path the Parkway takes before you actually cycle it. Where the Parkway cuts alongside Bluff Mountain, water trickles down gray-black rock that extends 50 feet up from the side of the road. It's fun to imagine what that same rock looks like in January after a few long, hard freezes. Through the winter months, the entire side of the mountain is covered in glimmering ice, inches thick.

Once out of the park, the road makes a rapid descent toward Laurel Springs. There are several miles of level cycling on the way to Laurel Springs, which is a touristy dot on the map with a few good facilities and some not-so-good facilities. Miller's Campground is located roughly 1 mile before Laurel Springs.

Once past Laurel Springs, the Parkway climbs again. The terrain is basically rolling mountain with a few hills you can actually crest without shifting down.

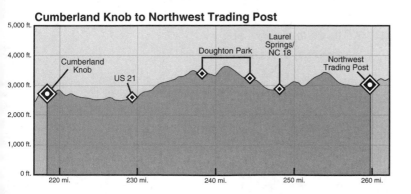

Cumberland Knob to Northwest Trading Post

If you enjoy checking out the local culture, Glendale Springs is the real treat of this area. The Church of the Frescoes and Glendale Springs Inn & Restaurant lend quaint charm to this community. Inside the Church of the Frescoes are life-size paintings, including *The Lord's Supper* and other religious scenes. A sunny country garden filled with zinnias, daylilies, poppies, and daisies surrounds the church. There is also an elaborate herb garden centered on two harps in town. One of these is an aeolian harp designed to be played by the wind.

The Northwest Trading Post is a co-op for North Carolina craftsmen. You must stop here, even if you do not venture into Glendale Springs. The Trading Post is crammed with quilts and other handcrafted items, such as lampshades decorated with pressed wildflowers, knitted afghans and sweaters, and wind chimes. The various homemade baked goods are delicious. There are country ham biscuits, hummingbird cake, molasses stack cake, peanut butter and oatmeal cookies, German chocolate cake, hoop cheese, dried apples, and more.

With camping, lodging, and so much to see, you might want to plan to make an early day of it here.

MILEPOST

218.6   FOX HUNTERS PARADISE (elevation 2,805')
This overlook has excellent views of the Piedmont.

229.7   US 21 (elevation 2,700')
Sparta, North Carolina
Sparta is 7 miles north on US 21. This well-traveled road has truck traffic and no shoulder. There are a few big hills coming into Sparta. If you want a diversion or you need special services, this may be a good time to divert off the Parkway. Sparta has banks, laundry facilities, a hospital, and a hardware store.

Alleghany Inn   336-372-2501 $–$$
Through town on US 21; open year-round.

230.1   LITTLE GLADE MILL POND (elevation 2,709')

232.5   VIEW OF STONE MOUNTAIN

238.5   BRINEGAR CABIN   336-372-8877
Historic cabin open for weekend tours; closed in winter.

238.6   DOUGHTON PARK [closed for 2014]
Announces itself long before any facilities are encountered. There is an excellent 12-mile trail system here.

239.2   DOUGHTON PARK CAMPGROUND   336-372-8877
This National Park Service campground is separated
from the restaurant and lodge by 2 steep miles. A
hiking trail connects the two facilities. There are 110
tent sites and 25 trailer sites in the campground,
though some loops may be closed.

241.1   BLUFFS LODGE AND COFFEE SHOP   336-372-4744
$$–$$$ [closed for 2014]
Coffee shop hours: daily, 7:30 a.m.–7:30 p.m. The
lodge, located on the east side, is open May–October.

244.8   DOUGHTON PARK
Southern boundary of Doughton Park

247.2   MILLER'S CAMPGROUND   336-359-8156
Visible on the west side, Miller's Campground is open
April–November. Facilities include showers, laundry,
ice, and a camp store.

248.0   NC 18 (elevation 2,851')
Laurel Springs, North Carolina

Laurel Springs is visible to the right of the Parkway, traveling south.

Freeborne's Eatery & Lodge   336-359-8008; freebornes.com $–$$
Motel, cottages, restaurant, and bar.

Wild Woody's Campground and Antique Store 336-359-8432 $

Mountain Side Campground   336-359-8487; mountainsidecampground.com [closed]
Campsites and log cabins available, but it's a steep 1.3-mile climb to the campground. At press time the site was closed due to change in ownership. Call ahead of time to make sure it's operating again.

256.0   MOUNTAIN VIEW LODGE AND CABINS 336-207-7677; mtnviewlodge.com $$–$$$
Located on the east side. Options include one- and two-bedroom cabins with kitchenettes. Breakfast is served in the lodge.

257.6   RACCOON HOLLER CAMPGROUND   336-982-2706; raccoonholler.com
Located on the west side of the Parkway, just north of Glendale Springs. Facilities include showers, laundry, and a camp store with grocery items.

259.0   GLENDALE SPRINGS—TRADING POST ROAD
Northwest Trading Post   336-982-2543
Open May–October, the Trading Post has home-made crafts and baked goods made by North Carolina craftsmen.

Glendale Springs, North Carolina
There is very little indication from the Parkway of the bounty that is Glendale Springs. This is a perfect example of what can lie just yards beyond the Parkway. Turn right and head south at the Northwest Trading Post.

**Church of the Frescoes   336-982-3076;
churchofthefrescoes.com**
In the center of town; fresco art includes *The Lord's
Supper, Mary Great With Child,* and *St. John the
Baptist.*

**Greenhouse Crafts Shop   336-982-2618;
greenhousecrafts.com**
Crafts, collectibles, books, stationery, and music.

Blue Ridge Bakery Café   336-982-4811
The only restaurant remaining in Glendale Springs
with sandwiches, salads, burgers, and baked goods.

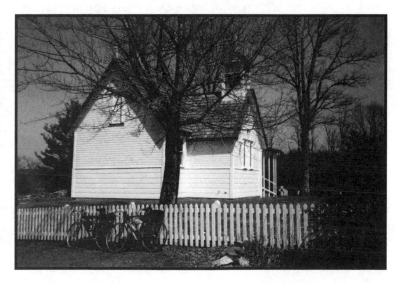

*A sunny country garden and white picket fence surround the
Church of the Frescoes.*

Northwest Trading Post to Linville Falls
[259–317]

There is no level ground from the trading post to Julian Price Memorial Park. You climb from the Northwest Trading Post, descend some, and then climb some more. You are headed toward Boone, Blowing Rock, and Grandfather Mountain, so higher elevations and the climbs that accompany them are inevitable.

There are several fine overlooks in this area, so at least cruise through them: view from the Lump (Milepost 264.4), Mount Jefferson Overlook (Milepost 266.9), and Elk Mountain Overlook (Milepost 274.3). At E. B. Jeffress Park a brief trail leads to Cascades Waterfall.

In the 37 miles between the Northwest Trading Post and Julian Price, the Parkway takes you through a busy area. Those traveling south are approaching a spectacular section of the Parkway. Boone and Blowing Rock are major tourist areas. Blowing Rock is far more accessible to the Parkway than Boone. It has numerous motels with a wide price range and several excellent restaurants. Boone does offer one item that Blowing Rock lacks: a bike shop–several, in fact. While Boone is a great town, it is not necessary to travel that far since Blowing Rock is nearby. However, there is a fun way into Boone via Flannery Fork Road if you are traveling on a mountain bike or have tires tough enough to withstand several miles of gravel road. See our directions that follow.

To be sure, this is a great area for mountain bikes. At Moses H. Cone Memorial Park more than 20 miles of carriage paths wander around the estate. Moses H. Cone is a grand estate with a stately manor house perched on a hilltop that looks down on a man-made lake. The house and estate were donated to the National Park Service. The carriage trails are used for hiking, horseback riding, and cross-country skiing. Although these trails

Enjoy views of Price Lake from a lakeside campsite at Julian Price Park.

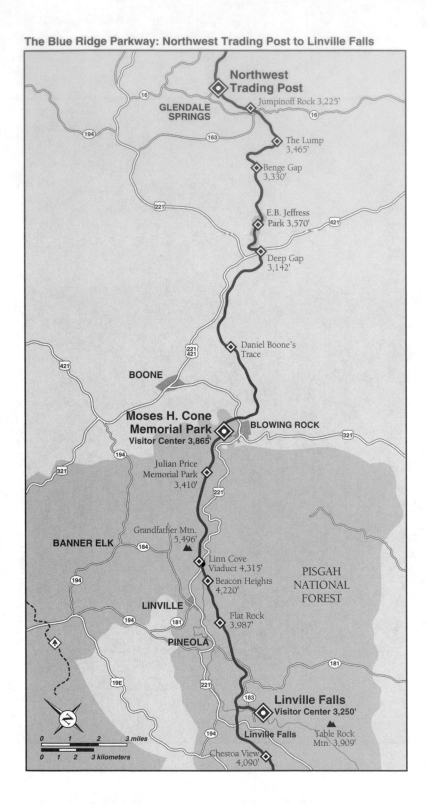

would be ideal for mountain biking, the official policy is a firm ban on bikes. The manor house is used as a gift shop for mountain crafts and pottery. The handicrafts here are very fine and come with expensive price tags. A vast array of pottery and hand-blown glassware, scarves and shawls made of fine wools, quilted clothing, and funky jewelry make you wish for more room in your bike bags.

At Julian Price Memorial Park you will want to be sure to get a campsite along Price Lake. If you have the time, you might want to fish for some rainbow trout or rent a canoe to go exploring. A hike around the lake after a full day of cycling would be a good way to work out the kinks. If you do camp at Julian Price, you can find food just 1.5 miles south of the campground on the access road to US 221.

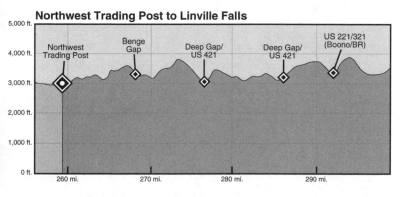

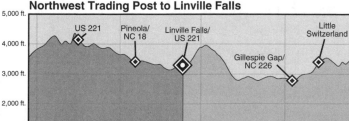

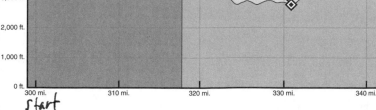

For the next 9 miles south of Julian Price Campground, the massive, 5,837-foot broad mountain known as Grandfather Mountain is ever present, watching over the entire Boone and Blowing Rock area. Before you get to Grandfather Mountain, you will encounter an engineering masterpiece–the Linn Cove Viaduct. Cycling across the Linn Cove Viaduct is a real thrill.

The viaduct winds around Grandfather Mountain in partial suspension. The road was built away from the mountain with supports underneath. As you cycle across, you can see streams that flow underneath the viaduct and can almost reach out and touch hemlocks and rhododendrons. Rather than whizzing past, on to your next destination, you can gain a finer appreciation of the vegetation of the area and the construction of the viaduct by hiking at least part of the trail that runs parallel to the viaduct.

The viaduct is not a difficult ride. The toughest part of this section is the unrelenting 5 miles preceding the Linn Cove Viaduct. It doesn't look all that bad, but the grade is considerable.

Once past the viaduct, you may want to stop at the Grandfather Mountain Overlook to reflect on what you have just passed through. If you are traveling north, the view as you approach Grandfather is spectacular.

Grandfather Mountain is an excellent side trip off the Parkway. Privately owned, the land is protected as a natural habitat for black bears, deer, and other wildlife. At the top of the mountain, there are picnic areas, a gift shop and restaurant, and the famous suspension bridge. As you stand in the middle of the bridge, you can feel the wind's destructive power. Winds on top of Grandfather have been known to gust well past 100 miles per hour.

Pineola is the next town of note just off the Parkway, with restaurants, a motel, campground, and a post office. From Pineola, the Parkway levels out for 4–5 miles into a straightaway. The presence of these level stretches always amazes us, especially in the midst of such mountainous terrain.

You are now approaching the Linville Gorge Wilderness Area. You could spend weeks hiking this wild, rugged area. If you are on a mountain bike, the U.S. Forest Service roads that circle the gorge are some of the steepest we have ever cycled. From the campground at Linville Falls, it is well worth a hike to the upper and lower falls. There are views of the gorge and the surrounding Linville Mountain, Hawksbill Mountain, Table Rock, and Jonas Ridge, composed of quartzite, and you are amid a geological history that goes back to the dinosaur days.

The Linville River attracts fly fishermen to this visitor center and campground. The river runs alongside the campsites on one side of the campground.

MILEPOST

268.0   BENGE GAP (elevation 3,330')

271.9   E. B. JEFFRESS PARK (elevation 3,570')
This park is primarily a picnic area with drinking water and restrooms. Cascades Nature Trail is a 0.6-mile hike to the falls.

276.4   DEEP GAP—US 421 (elevation 3,142')
It is 1 mile toward Boone to several convenience stores. US 421 is a heavily traveled two-lane road. We do not advise going into Boone this way.

286.9   US 421
EASTERN CONTINENTAL DIVIDE (elevation 3,100')
No facilities.

291.9   US 221 AND US 321

Blowing Rock, North Carolina

Two good routes lead into Blowing Rock, depending on the direction you are traveling. If you are heading south, take US 321 toward Blowing Rock and turn right onto US 321 Business. This is an easy ride into town. For those traveling north, take the US 221 exit before Moses H. Cone Memorial Park. It is a leisurely ride back and forth from Julian Price Memorial Path by this route. Dining and lodging possibilities abound in Blowing Rock. For more information on accommodations and dining, call the Blowing Rock Tourism Development Authority at 877–750–4636 or go to **blowingrock.com.** While there is no bike shop in Blowing Rock, Footsloggers is an excellent outdoor retailer with outdoor apparel and hiking equipment.

Boone, North Carolina

Boone is accessible by two routes. The first is via US 321; it is 7 miles north on this four-lane highway. Road conditions are fairly good due to the spaciousness of the road, but traffic can be aggravated during heavy tourist seasons. There is some downhill into Boone and, likewise, a fair amount of climbing back to the Parkway. The other way in is via Flannery Fork Road, for which there are signs just off the Parkway at Milepost 294.6. This road takes you right into the center of Boone. There are a couple of miles of rough gravel road, but the road is paved at least halfway. As in Blowing Rock, there are numerous dining and lodging possibilities in Boone. For detailed information on dining and lodging in Boone, call 828–264–1299 or go to **exploreboonearea.com.**

Alpen Acres Motel   888-297-7981, 828-295-7981; alpenacres.com $–$$

Conveniently located on the left, the motel is 0.2 mile north of the Parkway on US 321.

Boone Bike & Touring Co.   828-262-5750; boonebike.com
This bike shop is located at 774 E King St. (US 221).

Magic Cycles Inc.   828-265-2211; magiccycles.com
Take US 321 into town, turn left on US 421, and then
turn left onto Depot Street. Located at 140 S Depot
St. behind Farmers Hardware.

294.0   MOSES H. CONE MEMORIAL PARK (elevation 3,865')

294.6   US 221—2 miles into Blowing Rock
Flannery Fork Road is just off this exit.

296.4   PRICE PARK PICNIC AREA

296.9   JULIAN PRICE MEMORIAL PARK (elevation 3,410')
Price Campground
Julian Price has lakeside campsites and fishing. The
campground has 129 tent sites and 62 trailer sites.

298.6   US 221/HOLLOWAY MOUNTAIN ROAD
Exiting left on this road will take you to US 221, which
was the official Parkway route before the viaduct was
completed. A few stores are less than a mile down
Holloway, an easy trip on a bike from Price Campground.

Grandfather Country Store   828-295-6100;
grandfathercountrystore.com
At the intersection of Holloway Mountain Road and
US 221, this store has a good selection of groceries.
Lunch is served here also. Open year-round,
Thursday–Sunday, 11:30 a.m.–6 p.m.

304.4   LINN COVE VIADUCT INFORMATION CENTER
(elevation 4,315')
This visitor center and comfort station was built to accommodate the popularity of the Linn Cove Viaduct. The

Tanawha Trail begins here. Facilities include restrooms, telephones, and a gift shop. A ranger is on duty.

305.1   GRANDFATHER MOUNTAIN—US 221

Take US 221 to the right and proceed 3 miles to Grandfather Mountain. Privately owned and operated, facilities are open daily, April 1–November 15, and on winter days, weather permitting. Admission is $20 for adults, $9 for children ages 4–12. The road to the summit is extremely steep. For more information, call 800–468–7325; **grandfather.com.**

312   PINEOLA—NC 181

A spur road leads to NC 181, which leads right 1.6 miles into Pineola. There is a slight descent into town. You will find restaurants, a post office, and accommodations there.

Christa's Country Corner
This well-stocked grocery is open year-round and has a deli. Located right off the exit.

Pineola Inn & Country Store   828-733-4979; ktti.com/pineolainn $–$$
Located 1 mile from the Parkway.

Down by the River Family Campground   828-733-5057; downbytherivercampground.com
Mostly trailer sites with hookups; also 16 tent-only sites.

316.3   LINVILLE FALLS VISITOR CENTER

An easy, 1.5-mile road leads to parking and access to the Linville River and gorge as well as water and restrooms. A picnic area is located just off the Parkway.

Linville Falls Campground (elevation 3,250')
828-765-7818
Go 0.5 mile and look for the campground on the right, which has 55 tent sites and 20 trailer sites. Open year-round.

317.4   LINVILLE FALLS—US 221

Linville Falls has several motels and restaurants. The Linville Gorge Wilderness Area entrance is 3 miles off the Parkway, from US 221 onto NC 183, just beyond town.

Parkview Lodge & Cabins   800-849-4452, 828-765-4787; parkviewlodge.com $$

Just 0.2 mile south of the Parkway on US 221.

Linville Falls Lodge & Cottages   800-634-4421, 828-765-2658; linvillefallslodge.com $$–$$$

This motel is 0.5 mile south of the Parkway on US 221. Open April–November.

Linville Falls Trailer Lodge and Campground 828-765-2681; linvillefalls.com

Go 0.2 mile south on US 211, and then turn right on Gurney Franklin Road and go 1 mile.

Spear's BBQ and Grill   868-765-2658

Go south on US 211 for 0.7 mile. On left across from post office. Great North Carolina barbecue!

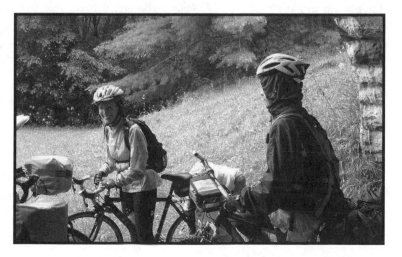

Cyclists take cover beneath a bridge near Pineola.

Linville Falls to Craggy Gardens [317–364]

Linville Falls and Crabtree Meadows are both wonderful areas from which to make day trips. You could set up base camp at either place and have plenty of options for exploring by bicycle. The various motels in Little Switzerland all make wonderful weekend getaways.

One of the highlights of this area is the vast apple orchard between Mileposts 328 and 329. In the fall, you can buy quite an assortment of apples, including Stayman Winesap, Stark Delicious, and York Imperial. If you are lucky enough to cycle through here between late April and early May, the apple blossoms will intoxicate you with their perfume.

NC 226 intersects the Parkway at Milepost 331. A side trip to Spruce Pine may not be necessary, but you can find grocery stores, restaurants, motels, and banks there. The Museum of North Carolina Minerals is located at this intersection. Time spent with the exhibits will give you an appreciation of the geology and mineralogy of the Blue Ridge. Displays of amethyst, quartz, emerald, mica, and other rocks and minerals native to the Blue Ridge explain the fascination that rock hounds have with the area.

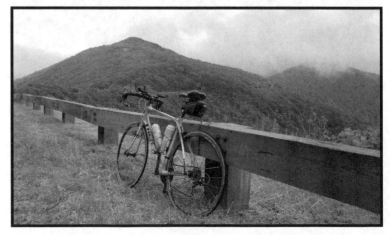

Approaching Craggy Gardens—a long climb from the north or the south

Little Switzerland is a pleasant side trip right off the Parkway at Milepost 334. There are three excellent motels here. This is a good place to treat yourself. Beyond this point heading south, there are very few accommodations until you reach Asheville. If you like to browse in shops, there are several good ones in Little Switzerland.

Little Switzerland Tunnel is the first of many tunnels from here to Cherokee. You may want to mount a lighting system from here on out. If nothing else, a flashing belt beacon on your rear will alert cars to your presence.

Crabtree Meadows has a campground, a restaurant, and a camp store. These are the last facilities on the Parkway proper until Mount Pisgah, which is 70 tough miles away. We recommend getting a motel room in Asheville so you can get cleaned up and fresh for the grueling climb from Asheville to Mount Pisgah.

Enjoy the fantastic descent you get in this section. From Chestoa View, elevation 4,090 feet, you will drop down to 2,819 feet at Gillespie Gap. That's almost 10 miles of pure downhill. From Gillespie Gap you will begin a climb into the Black Mountains, which culminates with Mount Mitchell at 6,684 feet.

Speaking of Mount Mitchell, just how big of a deal can one mountain be? Just ask anyone who has done the annual Assault on Mount Mitchell. If you are undertaking the Parkway in a big way, you owe it to yourself to cycle to the top of Mount Mitchell. You don't want to deny yourself the opportunity of being able to say you've cycled up to the highest peak east of the Mississippi River. The gain in elevation on the 4.8-mile spur road to the summit is 1,390 feet. The view is unparalleled. The descent is nerve-tingling. The damage to the spruce and fir forests by the woolly aphid and acid rain should be witnessed. Motorists will think you are crazy, but Mount Mitchell is a bicyclist's mecca.

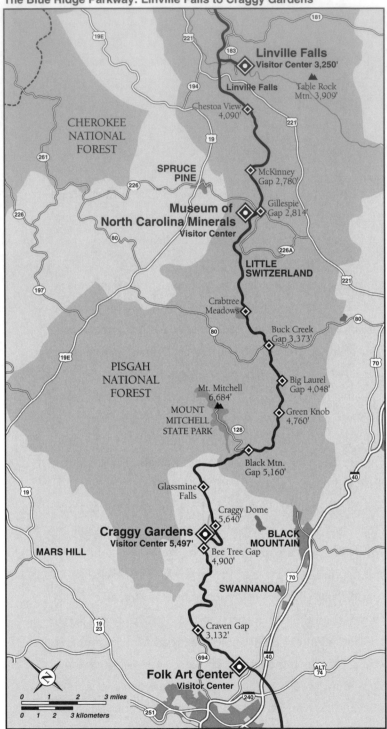

For those wondering what the Assault on Mount Mitchell is all about, it's a 102-mile endurance event open to anyone crazy enough to try it. Sponsored by the Spartanburg Freewheelers, the event begins in Spartanburg, South Carolina, in late May. In recent years the number of riders has been limited to 800, the maximum number allowed on the Parkway by the National Park Service and Mount Mitchell State Park. For more information, contact the Freewheelers at 800-636-6773, ext. 6664, or go to the group's website at **freewheelers.info.**

Camping at Mount Mitchell State Park allows you a chance to experience the harsh weather conditions characteristic of the higher elevations. These campsites are not fully exposed, but they are situated on the side of the mountain. Mist or rain is likely. The gusting winds characteristic of the mountain are sure to whip

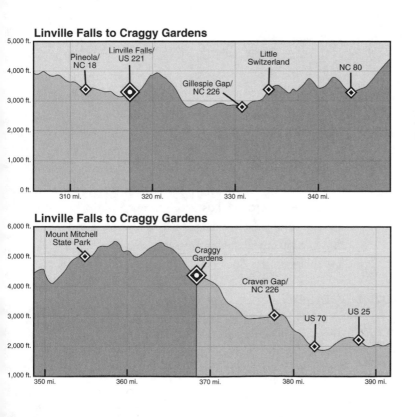

your little nylon tent all through the night. There are only nine sites here and they are fairly primitive. Don't expect asphalt leading up to your tent pad. Arrive before noon to get one of these precious sites.

The Parkway is spectacular from Mount Mitchell to Craggy Gardens. You are in the midst of the Black Mountains, and they deliver. This entire area is a cyclist's dream. Granted, you have to work extremely hard, but that always serves to heighten the experience. We would feel cheated if we drove in a car through this area. Once you've traveled the Parkway on a bike, you won't want to do it any other way.

Craggy Gardens is known for its rhododendrons. Hiking trails take you to the top of the bald, where the view of the Black Mountains is supreme. In addition to rhododendrons, mountain laurels, blueberries, mountain cranberries, and mountain ash exist in abundance. Mountain ash grab your attention in the late fall, after the leaves have fallen, when their brilliant red berries provide the only bright color.

MILEPOST

324.8   BEAR DEN CAMPGROUND
828-765-2888; bear-den.com

Be on the lookout for Bear Den Mount Road on the east side of the Parkway. A moderately steep, rough-paved 0.6-mile road leads to the campground. This campground is well managed with showers, laundry, and a camp store. Cabins are available year-round; 144 tent sites are open March–November.

328.1   ALTA PASS

The Orchard at Alta Pass   828-765-9531, 888-765-9531; altapassorchard.org

Located on the east side, this store has souvenirs, ice cream, and light snacks. Music, hayrides, and more.

Open May–October: Monday and Wednesday–
Saturday, 10 a.m.–5 p.m.; Sunday, noon–5 p.m.

331.0   GILLESPIE GAP—NC 226 (elevation 2,814')
Museum of North Carolina Minerals   828-765-2761
Located right off the Parkway, this National Park Service museum features excellent exhibits of area
rocks and minerals. A bookstore, restrooms, and
drinking water are available. NC 226 intersects here.
You can take a back way into Little Switzerland via
NC 226A. If you turn left and go under the bridge, you
will find a motel and convenience store. Open daily,
9 a.m.–5 p.m.

Pine Valley Motel   828-765-6276;
pinevalleymotel.com $$
About 3.5 miles from the Parkway going north on NC
226. Open year-round.

Spruce Pine, North Carolina
Spruce Pine is a whopping 6 miles from the Parkway
going north on NC 226. There are two major grocery
stores, a drugstore, a hardware store, banks, and
restaurants.

Skyline Village Inn & Cavern Tavern   828-765-9394;
skylinevillageinn.com $
Located east of the Parkway on NC 226A.

Mountain View Restaurant   828-766-9670;
mountainviewrest.com
From the Parkway, take NC 226 beneath tunnel.
Located on right.

333.4   LITTLE SWITZERLAND TUNNEL (542 feet)

334.0   LITTLE SWITZERLAND, NORTH CAROLINA—NC 226A
Maybe call it an early day and hang out for the afternoon.

Sunrise view of Table Rock from Little Switzerland

Alpine Inn   828-765-5380; alpineinnnc.com $–$$
This motel is the farthest from the Parkway, but it is
dear to our hearts. It has the most reasonable rates
too. Turn right onto NC 226A and travel south 1 mile;
steep return to the Parkway. Open late April–early
November.

**Big Lynn Lodge   828-765-4257, 800-654-5232;
biglynnlodge.com $$$**
Visible on the east side of the Parkway. A hearty din-
ner and breakfast are included in the price. From the
Parkway exit, turn left on NC 226A and go about 1
mile. Open April–October.

**Switzerland Inn   828-765-2153, 800-654-4026;
switzerlandinn.com $–$$$**
Located on the left immediately off the Parkway, this
elegant lodge was established in 1910. For the econ-
omy minded, the inn has a bunkhouse with eight
rooms connected to a central living room. Breakfast

for two is included. If you prefer a little pampering, stay at the inn proper. Wonderful views of the valley lie below.

Switzerland Café and General Store   828-765-5289; switzerlandcafe.com
On the way to the Alpine Inn, you can stop here for gourmet deli sandwiches.

336.8   WILDACRES TUNNEL (330 feet)

339.5   CRABTREE MEADOWS [closed for 2014]
Crabtree Meadows has 71 tent sites and 22 trailer sites. Crabtree Falls is a 40-minute walk from the campground.

Crabtree Meadows Coffee Shop   828-675-4236 [closed for 2014]
Coffee shop and camp store stocked with basic grocery items. We just wish that the food counter opened earlier for breakfast. With a strenuous 5-mile round-trip to Mount Mitchell ahead for southbounders, breakfast is a must. Restaurant hours: May–October: daily, 9:30 a.m.–6 p.m.

340.2   CRABTREE MEADOWS PICNIC AREA   [closed for 2014]
Has water and restrooms.

344.0   NC 80 (elevation 3,373')
There are just a few recommended facilities within close range of this intersection.

Carolina Hemlocks Recreation Area   828-675-5509
This Pisgah National Forest campground has a bracing mountain stream that feeds a deep swimming pool, but it is 6 miles north toward Burnsville. Cycling to Carolina Hemlocks from Crabtree Meadows or Little Switzerland and back makes an outstanding day trip.

Jewell's Mt. Mitchell View Restaurant   828-675-9214
Located 1.5 miles north on NC 80; a very steep
descent and return. Monday–Saturday, 11 a.m.–7 p.m.

344.5   TWIN TUNNEL (NORTH) (300 feet)

344.7   TWIN TUNNEL (SOUTH) (401 feet)

349.0   ROUGH RIDGE TUNNEL (150 feet)

355.4   MOUNT MITCHELL STATE PARK

The road to the summit is a 5-mile climb with grades reaching 8%. This is much steeper than any other grade on Skyline Drive or the Parkway. Actually, the first 2 miles to the summit are steeper than the last 3. There's a snack bar, natural history museum, and observation tower at the top. The campground is 4 miles from the Parkway. Remember, there are only nine campsites and they are first come, first served. There is a restaurant here also, but it sometimes closes during the peak season. Open May–October. Restaurant hours: Monday–Friday, 11 a.m.–8 p.m.; Saturday–Sunday, 8 a.m.–8 p.m.

361.2   VIEW OF GLASSMINE FALLS

A 0.1-mile trail leads to a view of this 800-foot falls.

364.1   CRAGGY DOME PARKING OVERLOOK (elevation 5,640')

364.4   CRAGGY PINNACLE TUNNEL (245 feet)

364.4   CRAGGY GARDENS (elevation 5,497')

Craggy Gardens has a visitor center with restrooms, drinking water, and a good selection of literature on the Blue Ridge. Take a hike to Craggy Dome, Craggy Pinnacle, and Craggy Knob.

367   BEE TREE GAP—CRAGGY GARDENS PICNIC AREA

It has 86 sites plus restrooms, and it's wheelchair accessible.

Craggy Gardens to Mount Pisgah [364–406]

Get ready for some fun. You have a solid 10 miles of spectacular downhill into Asheville. You'll gain it back if you are cycling on to Mount Pisgah, but for now, enjoy. Pisgah National Forest spreads its lush blanket of green as far as the eye can see. The Swannanoa River Valley and the town of Black Mountain are to the east.

Known as The Land of the Sky, Asheville is the quintessential city of the Blue Ridge. With a metropolitan population of 425,000, it has become an urban center in its own right. Its burgeoning size warrants some careful directions on how to get around. We suggest that you take one of two routes to reach the inner city. Town Mountain Road leads to downtown Asheville and two bike shops. The route through Biltmore Forest situates you best for the Biltmore Estate. A third route is best for reaching the airport. We outline each route below.

Of modern design in wood and stone, the Folk Art Center sits serenely in its mountain setting. If you appreciate fine handicrafts, you will want several hours to spend here. Bring your credit card because the artsy jewelry, handloomed fabrics, and original pottery are expensive. The Folk Art Center also has an extensive selection of books on the Southern Highlands.

There are numerous tourist attractions in Asheville. The Biltmore Estate, the Thomas Wolfe Memorial and home, and the seasonal festivals held in Asheville are all reasons to spend some time in the city. If you plan on touring Asheville, you may want to visit the Asheville Convention & Visitors Bureau website, **exploreasheville.com,** for detailed information.

Past Asheville, over a 12-mile section between Milepost 397 and 409, you'll encounter nine tunnels, ranging in length from 275 to 1,320 feet. Pine Mountain Tunnel at Milepost 399.1 is the longest on the Parkway. Let your imagination run wild with the names of

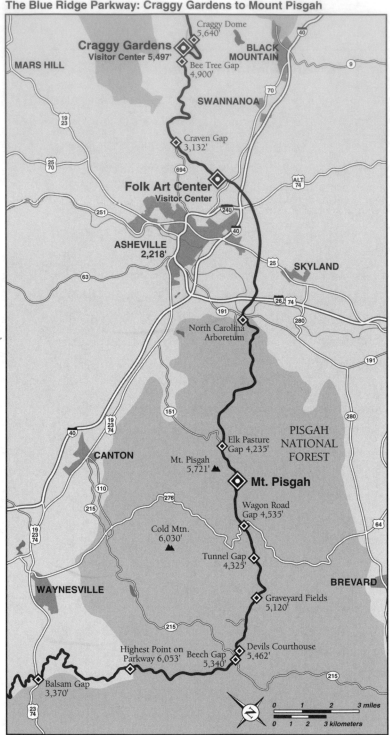

The Blue Ridge Parkway: Craggy Gardens to Mount Pisgah

Craggy Dome
5,640'

BLACK
MOUNTAIN

Craggy Gardens
Visitor Center 5,497'

MARS HILL

Bee Tree Gap
4,900'

SWANNANOA

Craven Gap
3,132'

Folk Art Center
Visitor Center

ASHEVILLE
2,218'

SKYLAND

North Carolina
Arboretum

Elk Pasture
Gap 4,235'

PISGAH
NATIONAL
FOREST

CANTON

Mt. Pisgah
5,721'

Mt. Pisgah

Wagon Road
Gap 4,535'

Cold Mtn.
6,030'

Tunnel Gap
4,325'

BREVARD

WAYNESVILLE

Graveyard Fields
5,120'

Highest Point on
Parkway 6,053'

Beech Gap
5,340'

Devils Courthouse
5,462'

Balsam Gap
3,370'

0   1   2   3 miles

0   1   2   3 kilometers

the tunnels as you travel through them: Buck Spring, Ferrin Knob, Grassy Knob, Young Pisgah Ridge, Fork Mountain . . . you'll need the diversion with all of the climbing you've got to do. From Milepost 384 to Milepost 408, you will climb 3,705 feet. You may have to get off your bike and cry, but you'll make it. This is why Asheville is such a good break point for cyclists doing extended tours. Whether you are traveling north or south, you will have a climb out of Asheville. Take heart if you are touring the Parkway north to south. The climb from Asheville to Mount Mitchell is worse, at a grand total of 4,265 feet climbed to the entrance of Mount Mitchell State Park.

At Milepost 399.7 you might want to stop and view Pisgah Ridge rising up to the 5,749-foot peak of Mount Pisgah. You will be traveling across Pisgah Ridge because the Parkway follows it for 24 miles to Tanasee Bald. At Tanasee Bald the Parkway enters the Great Balsam Range.

The historic presence of the Vanderbilts is evident upon reaching Mount Pisgah. In the late 1800s, George Washington Vanderbilt bought 130,000 acres of land in the area, including Mount Pisgah. Remnants of a stone foundation are all that are left of Vanderbilt's mountain retreat at Buck Spring Gap.

Pisgah Inn is truly a mountain retreat. It hugs the side of the mountain, and the floor-to-ceiling picture windows in the dining

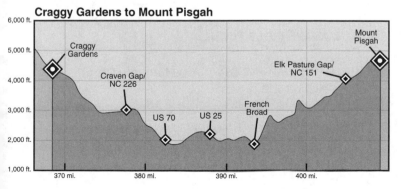

room and each of the guest rooms frame views of the hazy blue ridges toward Hendersonville and Brevard. Pisgah Inn is the place to sample rainbow trout, prepared here five different ways.

Camping here is enjoyable; with an excellent store and restaurant dining as an option, you have plenty of resources at your disposal. A day or two spent here is full of possibilities. The steep hike to the magnificent Mount Pisgah can occupy an entire afternoon. There's a weather station and an observation tower at the summit. It's windy at the top, and weather changes can be sudden, so bring a jacket. Additional hikes, in all directions from the campground, make for plenty of exploring.

Mountain laurels and several varieties of rhododendrons, including catawba, Carolina, and rosebay, are abundant in the campground, as well as a couple miles farther in the Cradle of Forestry. An overlook at Milepost 410.3 reveals the Pink Beds, part of the Cradle of Forestry area of Pisgah National Forest, which are a dense undergrowth of mountain laurels and rosebay rhododendrons interspersed with tiny mountain bogs. Late May–June is the time to find the rhododendrons and laurels in bloom. Wildflowers are prolific all summer throughout the campground and the grounds surrounding the inn.

MILEPOST

365.5   CRAGGY FLATS TUNNEL (400 feet)

374.4   TANBARK RIDGE TUNNEL (780 feet)

377.4   CRAVEN GAP—NC 694 (Town Mountain Road)
(elevation 3,132')

Exiting the Parkway here places you in downtown Asheville and near several hotels, restaurants, and bike shops. Town Mountain Road is a two-lane scenic highway that winds through a residential area. (*Warning:*

There's no shoulder on this busy, narrow road.) From the Parkway, Town Mountain Road climbs for about 2 miles and then descends the mountain into Asheville. Be careful on the switchbacks on the steep descent into town. Turn right onto College Street, about 6.5 miles from the Parkway. At the second traffic light, turn right onto Oak Street, which turns almost immediately into Woodfin Street.

Hearn's Cycling & Fitness   828-253-4800
Follow Town Mountain Road route above, continuing on Woodfin Street to second light. Turn left and then right on ALT 74A. Turn left onto Asheland Avenue; shop is on the left. Hours: Monday–Saturday, 8:30 a.m.–5:30 p.m.

BioWheels   828-236-2453; biowheels.com
Follow Town Mountain Road route above, continuing on Woodfin Street to second light. Turn left. Turn right onto Hilliard Avenue, and take the fourth right onto Coxe Avenue. Shop is on the left. Hours: Tuesday–Friday, noon–6 p.m.; Saturday, noon–5 p.m.

Ski Country Sports   828-254-2771; skicountrysports.com
Follow Town Mountain Road route above, continuing on Woodfin Street to second light. Turn right onto Broadway, which soon turns into Merrimon Avenue. Go about 4 miles north to 1000 Merrimon Ave. Store is on the left. Hours: Monday–Saturday, 10 a.m.–6 p.m.

Pro Bikes of Asheville   828-253-2800; pro-bikes.com
This bike shop relocated several miles beyond downtown across the French Broad River to west Asheville at 610 Haywood Rd. Call for directions. Hours: Monday–Friday, 10 a.m.–7 p.m.; Saturday,

10 a.m.–5 p.m. (opens at 11 a.m. in January and February).

Four Points by Sheraton   828-253-1851 $$–$$$
Located on right at 22 Woodfin St.

Renaissance Hotel Asheville   828-252-8211 $$$
Located on left off Woodfin Street, across from Four Points by Sheraton.

382.0   FOLK ART CENTER   828-298-7928; **southernhighlandguild.org**
Operated by the Southern Highland Craft Guild, this is a required stop for anyone interested in crafts, books, or history and information on the Blue Ridge. Restrooms, drinking water, and snacks are available here.

382.5   US 70 INTERSECTION
The closest facilities are just 1 mile east on US 70 toward Black Mountain. There are numerous motels and several restaurants.

Motel 6   828-299-3040 $

Days Inn Biltmore East   828-298-4000 $–$$

Holiday Inn Biltmore East   828-298-5611 $$–$$$

Quality Inn & Suites Biltmore East
828-298-5519 $$–$$$
Heading west on US 70 toward Asheville, you will find a grocery store, post office, and banks. Asheville VA Medical Center is located 1.3 miles from the Parkway on US 70 West.

383.5   I-40 crosses underneath the Parkway (elevation 2,040')

384.7   US 74 INTERSECTION

Avoid this interchange. There is nothing here of note.

388.1   US 25

This is our recommended exit for the Asheville Regional
Airport and the most accessible bike shop in Asheville,
Liberty Bicycles. You can take US 25 into Asheville, but it
is a well-traveled, two-lane highway. There are major
shopping centers within 0.25 mile of the Parkway in
either direction on US 25.

Liberty Bicycles   828-274-2453; libertybikes.com

Take US 25 north 0.3 mile toward Asheville. Located in
a strip mall on the right by a major grocery store (1378
Hendersonville Rd.). Hours: Monday–Saturday,
10 a.m.–6 p.m.; Sunday, noon–5 p.m.

Asheville Regional Airport

Follow US 25 South (a four-lane highway) to Airport
Road. Turn right onto Airport Road and follow to the
airport. This entire area is congested.

Biltmore Estate   800-411-3812; biltmore.com

At the US 25 exit, we found a beautiful route into the
tourist area of Asheville. Biltmore Estate is only 4
miles via this route. On the way, you get to cycle
through one of the most elegant neighborhoods in
Asheville. Take the US 25 South exit and turn left into
Biltmore Forest. Take an immediate right onto
Stuyvesant Road. Follow this road about 2 miles until
it merges onto Vanderbilt Road. You will bear right
here. Vanderbilt Road ends at Hendersonville Road,
3.6 miles from the Parkway. Biltmore Estate is 0.25
mile to your left from the light. You are in the midst
of Biltmore Village, which has numerous gift shops.
There are several motels in the area. Admission to
the estate varies, but is typically about $50 for adults
and $25 for children.

DoubleTree Hotel   828-274-1800 $$$
Located at 115 Hendersonville Rd.

Quality Inn & Suites Biltmore South
828-684-6688 $$–$$$
The Quality Inn is at 1 Skyline Inn Dr.

Biltmore Howard Johnson Lodge   828-274-2300 $–$$
190 Hendersonville Rd.

Sleep Inn   828-277-1800 $–$$
117 Hendersonville Rd.

GuestHouse Inn & Suites   828-274-0101 $$–$$$
Located 3.2 miles north on US 25, 234 Hendersonville Rd.

393.6   FRENCH BROAD RIVER (elevation 2,000')
NC 191 intersects the Parkway here. There are picnic
areas along the river just off the Parkway in both directions. There are a few facilities on busy, four-lane NC 191
north with no major climbs. Biltmore Square Mall and a
Comfort Suites motel are 2.1 miles from the Parkway.

North Carolina Arboretum   828-665-2492;
ncarboretum.org
Several miles of trails wind through this wonderful
resource for learning about trees and plants. Open
year-round. No parking fee for bikes.

Carolina Fatz Cycling Center   828-665-7744;
carolinafatzmountainbicycle.com
This bike shop is 1.5 miles north on NC 191.
Open Monday–Saturday, 10 a.m.–6 p.m.

Comfort Suites   828-665-4000
This motel is 2.1 miles north on NC 191.

Lake Powhatan Recreation Area   828-670-5627
This Pisgah National Forest campground is quite a
detour from the Parkway. It's only 3 miles south on
NC 191 off the Parkway, but it's mostly downhill.

397.1   GRASSY KNOB TUNNEL (770 feet)

399.1   PINE MOUNTAIN TUNNEL (1,434 feet)
This is the longest tunnel on the Parkway.

400.9   FERRIN KNOB TUNNEL NO. 1 (561 feet)

401.3   FERRIN KNOB TUNNEL NO. 2 (421 feet)

401.5   FERRIN KNOB TUNNEL NO. 3 (375 feet)

403.0   YOUNG PISGAH RIDGE TUNNEL (412 feet)

404.0   FORK MOUNTAIN TUNNEL (389 feet)

404.7   ELK PASTURE GAP—NC 151 (elevation 4,235')

406.9   LITTLE PISGAH TUNNEL (576 feet)

407.3   BUCK SPRINGS TUNNEL (462 feet)

407.8   MOUNT PISGAH PICNIC AREA (elevation 4,900')

408.6   PISGAH INN   828-235-8228; pisgahinn.com $$$
Pisgah Inn's reputation precedes it. Reservations are
strongly suggested. At the very least, treat yourself

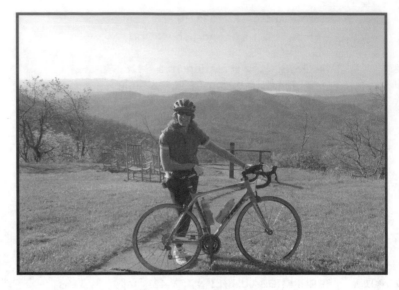

Views of Asheville from the back lawn at Pisgah Inn

to a meal here. You deserve it after your crazy cycling antics. You will also find telephones and a camp store here. Open April–October.

408.8   MOUNT PISGAH CAMPGROUND
(elevation 4,850')   **828-648-2644**
The campground is on the west side, near the Pisgah Inn. The campground has 70 tent sites and 70 trailer sites.

Mount Pisgah to Cherokee [409–469]

It is 60 rugged miles to Cherokee, and you had better be well prepared. Facilities are scarce in these parts. You will be cycling along Pisgah Ridge to the Great Balsams. You will reach the highest point on both Skyline Drive and the Blue Ridge Parkway at Richland Balsam, elevation 6,053 feet. Stop here and take it all in. You have truly come far if you have cycled from Front Royal to this point. It is a major achievement to get here from Cherokee or Asheville.

Awesome describes this section of the Parkway. From Mount Pisgah, the first geologic feature to command your attention is Looking Glass Rock. Its prominent, bare granite dome has become quite famous. After five or six preliminary miles of ups and downs, the Parkway begins the long ascent to Richland Balsam. Graveyard Fields and Graveyard Ridge are eerie in their barren, flat appearance described as boglike because of their lack of trees. In 1925 a forest fire destroyed 25,000 acres of spruce–fir forest. Today, the forest is slowly recovering: the "fields" are now filled with blueberries, mountain laurels, rhododendrons, and bush honeysuckle.

It could be argued that the best way to appreciate this area is by foot. Many areas of these mountains are accessible only by hiking trails. The Shining Rock Wilderness Area is 13,400 acres of wild mountain terrain. A spur road at Milepost 420.2 takes you to Ivestor Gap, where the hiking trails begin. You might have time to take a brief hike to the top of Devil's Courthouse, by way of the trail at Milepost 422.4, on your way to Cherokee. When mists hug this rocky, rugged summit, it looks devilish for sure.

The manner in which the trees grow in this section is something you can appreciate as you make the arduous climb to Richland Balsam. Fraser firs and red spruces are symbols of these mountains. They are the true inhabitants, able to survive the

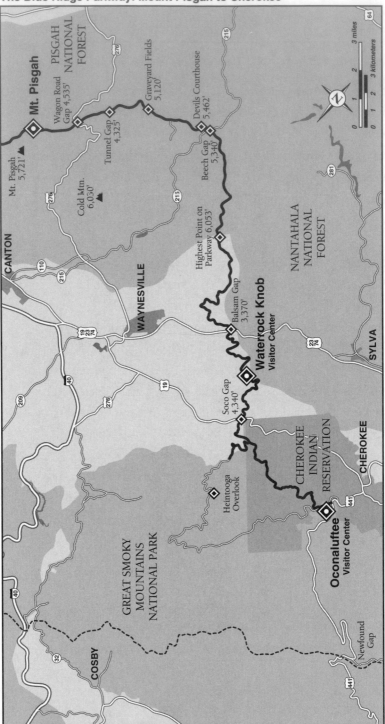

brutal climate of higher elevations. The one disturbing thing
about cycling through Richland Balsam is the sight of the dead
Fraser firs that cover the highest peaks. Just as with Mount Mitchell, the Fraser fir is dying because of an insect called the balsam
woolly aphid and other environmental stresses such as acid rain.
It is hoped that ultimately the Fraser fir will be able to genetically
adapt to this parasite.

Logic would follow that since you have just cycled to the
highest point on the Parkway, surely you will now have a great
descent. Well, you do. You also have a climb back up to Waterrock
Knob before the final descent into Cherokee. The grand total of
elevation climbed in this entire stretch is 6,225 feet. For those
cycling from Cherokee to Mount Pisgah, you will have to endure
a total climb of 9,305 feet. The major portion of this climb, 7,470
feet, is from Cherokee to Richland Balsam.

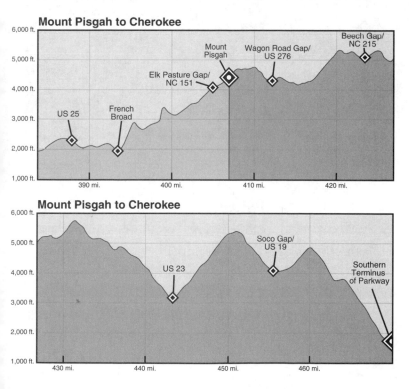

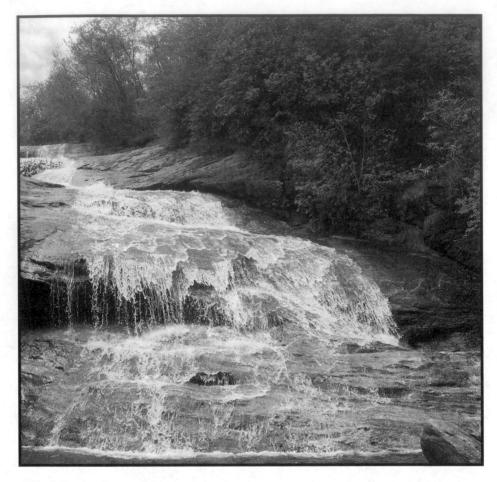

Waterfall at Devil's Courthouse

There has been some debate over which direction is tougher for cyclists, north to south or south to north. The general consensus is that the Parkway is tougher traveling south to north. In fact, the total feet climbed is higher in this direction, but not by much: 48,722 feet versus 48,601 feet. (See Appendix C for details.)

What options do you have if you can't cycle this section in a single day? Well, Balsam Mountain Campground isn't a lot of help. The spur road up to it climbs an additional 1,100 feet, and all you have left is a 10-mile descent into Cherokee. Your single alternative for lodging and food is the exit toward Waynesville at Balsam Gap, Milepost 443.1. This is an easy descent toward the town of Balsam, where you will find food, a motel, and a campground. Aside from this, the only feasible exit we know of is at Soco Gap. Any other way off the Parkway involves a major descent and too many miles detoured off the Parkway.

The descent into Cherokee is a cyclist's dream. Don't get carried away in the tunnels. They are much more dangerous when you are traveling at top speeds. There are six tunnels between Soco Gap and Cherokee.

MILEPOST

410.1   FRYING PAN TUNNEL (577 feet)

411.9   WAGON ROAD GAP—US 276 (elevation 4,535')
Cradle of Forestry in America Visitor Center
828-877-3130
It is a steep 4-mile descent from the Parkway on US 276 South. If your base camp is Mount Pisgah, this would be a good side trip. The visitor center has exhibits, a movie, and interpretive trails. Open daily, 9 a.m.–5 p.m. April–November. An entrance fee of $5 for age 16 and up is charged.

The Hub at Backcountry Outdoors   828-884-8670; thehubpisgah.com
This bike shop is in the town of Pisgah Forest, 15 miles from the Parkway on US 276 South. Open Monday–Friday, 10 a.m.–6 p.m.; Saturday, 9 a.m.–6 p.m.; Sunday, 10 a.m.–5 p.m.

422.1   DEVIL'S COURTHOUSE TUNNEL (665 feet)

423.3   BEECH GAP—NC 25 (elevation 5,340')

431.4   RICHLAND BALSAM OVERLOOK (elevation 6,053')
Highest point on the Blue Ridge Parkway.

439.7   PINNACLE RIDGE TUNNEL (813 feet)

443.1   BALSAM, NORTH CAROLINA—US 23/74
(elevation 3,370')

Balsam Mountain Inn   800-224-9498, 828-456-9498;
balsammountaininn.net $$$
Elegant accommodations located 1.7 miles from the
Parkway, complete with library, porches, great room,
country breakfast, lunch, and dinner. Go south on US
23/74. In between highway mile markers 93 and 94,
turn left on Candlestick Lane, and then make the
sharp right on Cabin Flats Drive. Follow road across
railroad tracks (twice). Located on hill on left.

451.2   WATERROCK KNOB PARKING OVERLOOK
(elevation 5,718')
You will find restrooms and drinking water here.

455.7   SOCO GAP—US 19 (elevation 4,340')
It is 5 miles straight down to Maggie Valley on a two-
lane highway.

458.2   BALSAM MOUNTAIN CAMPGROUND (elevation 5,240')
The campground at Balsam Mountain is part of Great
Smoky Mountains National Park. Take Heintooga
Spur Road 8.6 miles to the campground, with a gain
in elevation of 1,100 feet. There are 40 campsites
here. Facilities include drinking water and restrooms.
The campground may be closed, so call beforehand.

458.8   LICKSTONE RIDGE TUNNEL (402 feet)

459.3   BUNCHES BALD TUNNEL (255 feet)

461.2   BIG WITCH TUNNEL (348 feet)

465.6   RATTLESNAKE MOUNTAIN TUNNEL (395 feet)

466.2   SHERRIL COVE TUNNEL (550 feet)

469.1   END OF THE BLUE RIDGE PARKWAY (elevation 2,020')
For the record, the Parkway is actually 470 miles long. The Linn Cove Viaduct altered the total mileage. There are no immediate plans to change the mileposts.

Cherokee, North Carolina (elevation 2,020')
You are now connected with Great Smoky Mountains National Park. It is 2 miles south of Cherokee by way of US 441. There are numerous lodging possibilities.

Magnuson Hotel Great Smokies Inn
828-497-2020 $$$
Off Big Cove Road, 0.8 mile from the Parkway entrance.

Baymont Inn & Suites   828-497-2102 $$–$$$
Located 1 mile south of the Parkway on Acquoni Road.

Comfort Suites   828-497-3500 $$–$$$
Located about 1 mile south of the Parkway on US 441 South.

Cherokee KOA   828-497-9711
On US 441 South take the first left to Big Cove Road and follow signs 4 miles to campground. You'll find a pool and a camp store here.

Newfound Lodge   828-497-2746 $$
On the Oconaluftee River, located 1 mile from the Parkway entrance on US 441 North.

Riverside Motel & Campground   877-643-1439;
riversidemotelnc.com $$
Located 0.75 mile south of Cherokee on US 441. Waterfront rooms and campsites.

Great Smoky Mountains National Park

You can continue for 33 miles from Cherokee to Gatlinburg through Great Smoky Mountains National Park on US 441. The road is similar in character to the Parkway. The highest elevation on the road through the Smokies is 5,048 feet at Newfound Gap. The campgrounds in Great Smoky Mountains National Park have a reputation for filling up quickly, so arrive early. Gatlinburg is loaded with motels and restaurants.

Smokemont Campground   828-497-9270
Smokemont is just 3.8 miles from the southern terminus of the Parkway. Exit right onto US 441.

PART 3
Day Trips and Overnighters

While *Bicycling the Blue Ridge* is ultimately a guidebook for touring Skyline Drive and the Blue Ridge Parkway end-to-end, in reality, most cyclists experience these roads as life and schedules allow. Many of us have only the weekends to cycle. You can maximize a weekend experience by choosing sections wisely. Do keep in mind that the Parkway can have high traffic volume on weekends, especially around popular destinations such as the Asheville, Boone, and Roanoke areas. Overnighters are a great way to travel light, spend the night in an inn or bed-and-breakfast, and experience an area in more detail.

Cycling the Parkway on a racing bike is entirely different from a loaded touring bike. If you plan very carefully, you can carry an ultralight backpack, fanny pack, or hydration pack with essentials for an overnight trip. Rain or other inclement weather would be the main factor that could wreck an overnight trip, so a close watch on the forecast is important.

Another important consideration for an overnight trip is securing your vehicle. We advise parking in a National Park Service area such as a visitor center or campground and checking in with a ranger to let them know your car will be there overnight.

Destination Lodges on Skyline Drive and the Blue Ridge Parkway

Because several lodges are closed on the Parkway, the list on the following page includes the three remaining National Park Service lodges of note. Each is worth an overnight stay. The only tough aspect of each of these lodges is their relative mountaintop status–meaning tough climbs from either direction to them. One suggestion is to use them as a base and plan trips out and back from them. The other is to choose a starting point and cycle to them for an overnight stay.

❋ **Big Meadows** (Skyline Drive) has a rustic feel with a restaurant, hiking trails, and the namesake big meadow with acres of blueberries that attract a huge deer population.

❋ **Peaks of Otter** is newly remodeled in the picturesque setting of Abbott Lake and Sharp Top Mountain. It features a restaurant, bar, gift shop, walking trails, and scenic balcony rooms.

❋ **Pisgah Inn** hugs the side of the mountain south of Asheville and showcases amazing views of the Asheville valley and Pisgah National Forest. Hike to the top of Mount Pisgah and reward yourself with dinner; try the mountain trout prepared three ways.

Recommended Overnighters

MOUNT PISGAH TO CHEROKEE—63 MILES (difficult)

This is one of the most spectacular, rugged sections of the Parkway, and water, food, and facilities are sparse. You travel to the highest point on the Parkway at 6,053 feet. Traveling south you will climb 7,600 feet, descend 10,000 feet, and cycle through six tunnels. Simply awesome.

FOLK ART CENTER, ASHEVILLE TO LITTLE SWITZERLAND—48 MILES (difficult)

This trip is as thrilling and magnificent as the Pisgah/Cherokee section as it travels through Pisgah National Forest, past Mount Mitchell, and through the Black Mountains. The side trip to the top of Mount Mitchell is 5 additional miles. There are major climbs from the Folk Art Center to Craggy Gardens and Mount Mitchell. Jewell's Mt. Mitchell View Restaurant is a good lunch destination before you head into Little Switzerland. While small, Little Switzerland has shops and restaurants to explore. Two excellent inns–the Alpine Inn and the Switzerland Inn–offer breakfast and stunning views of the mountains from every room.

JULIAN PRICE PARK (BLOWING ROCK/BOONE) TO LITTLE SWITZERLAND—42 MILES (moderate)

The great reward of this section is cycling over the spectacular Linn Cove Viaduct, which is suspended and curves around Grandfather Mountain. Again, Little Switzerland is a pleasant overnight destination. You could reverse this and spend the night in Blowing Rock, which has numerous gift shops, restaurants, and motels.

NORTHWEST TRADING POST TO BLOWING ROCK —32 MILES (moderate)

This section is somewhat pastoral with plenty of ups and downs but no major climbs. Blowing Rock is easily accessible from the Parkway and has a wide variety of motels, shops, and restaurants.

MABRY MILL TO TUGGLE GAP (AND FLOYD, VA) —11 MILES plus 8 miles into Floyd on VA 8 (moderate)

Floyd, Virginia, is a laid-back mountain town with tasty cafés and artsy shops displaying pottery, jewelry, and other mountain crafts for sale. Floyd is a side trip off the Parkway, but it makes a nice

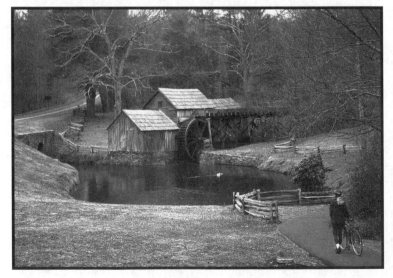

Mabry Mill is popular. The tour of the mill is fascinating!

diversion. Every summer, the town has a big music festival called Floyd Fest, as well as bluegrass jam sessions most every weekend.

ROCKY KNOB TO ROANOKE—49 MILES (moderate)

This is another pastoral section of the Parkway through the pretty Virginia countryside. In the summer, fields of wildflowers and crops make for pleasant cycling. See the point-by-point section for directions into Roanoke off the Parkway. Roanoke offers much to see and do.

ROANOKE TO PEAKS OF OTTER LODGE—34.4 MILES (moderate)

Both Roanoke and Peaks of Otter Lodge make excellent destinations, so try this day trip or overnighter either way depending on your interests. Peaks of Otter Lodge is newly renovated and offers a nice weekend retreat with scenic views and hiking trails from the lodge.

WAYNESBORO TO BIG MEADOWS LODGE—54.4 MILES (moderate)

FRONT ROYAL TO BIG MEADOWS—51 MILES (moderate)

At a midway point on Skyline Drive, Big Meadows Lodge is the perfect overnight destination. Skyline Drive climbs in both directions from Front Royal or Waynesboro to Big Meadows. Big Meadows has a rustic lodge with dining, a taproom, and a vast meadow that attracts deer at dusk and dawn.

Recommended Day Trips

Day trips can include any number of miles and any destinations you desire. The most significant aspect of day trips is transportation. Obviously, if you are limited to one vehicle, your trip will be out-and-back unless you do a loop off the Parkway. If you can bring two vehicles, parking a vehicle at each end is a great option. Over the years, we have done countless out-and-back day trips. Depending on your personality and your approach to cycling, the only problem with out-and-back day trips is getting hung up on elevation gained and lost. When you head out on the Parkway and come back the same route, you know full well what you have to climb to get back to your starting point. Ultimately there is something freeing about heading in one direction. You just take the Parkway and the elevation changes as they come.

All of the overnighter routes make excellent day trips. The main consideration is calculating the mileage you want to cover in one day and planning accordingly. Before you consider just 5 more miles, review the elevation profiles in the book and be aware of any major climbs in the section you have chosen.

We often plan day trips with a lunch destination as the halfway point. Some of the great destination points on the Parkway are closed due to the loss of a concessionaire to manage the facilities. As of this writing Crabtree Meadows and Doughton Park, both offering lunch options, are closed. Please check the Blue Ridge Parkway website, **nps.gov/blri,** before you plan a trip to make sure facilities are open.

CULTURAL AND HISTORICAL VISITOR CENTERS AROUND WHICH TO PLAN DAY TRIPS

* **Humpback Rocks Visitor Center and Farm** (exhibits and gift shop)
* **James River Visitor Center** (exhibit of the James River Canal)
* **Peaks of Otter Visitor Center** (exhibits and gift shop)
* **Mabry Mill** (mill exhibits, gift shop, and restaurant)
* **Blue Ridge Music Center** (no food but outstanding cultural exhibits)
* **Northwest Trading Post** (regional crafts, cheeses, baked goods, and beverages)

* **Moses H. Cone Memorial Park Visitor Center** (regional crafts)
* **Linn Cove Viaduct Visitor Center** (gift shop; Tanawha Trail meanders along the viaduct and leads to spectacular views from Grandfather Mountain)
* **Linville Falls Visitor Center** (exhibits and gift shop, but 1.4 miles off the Parkway)
* **Museum of North Carolina Minerals** (geological exhibits)
* **Mount Mitchell State Park** (visitor center, exhibits, trails, restaurant, and campground)
* **Craggy Gardens Visitor Center** (spectacular views and hiking trail)
* **Folk Art Center** (outstanding regional crafts and art)
* **Waterrock Knob Visitor Center** (gift shop and outstanding views)

continued on page 136

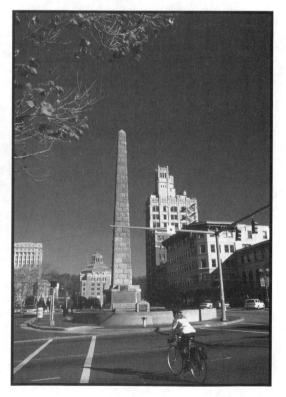

On an excursion into Asheville, this cyclist discovers City/County Park, site of many annual festivals as well as an obelisk dedicated to a Civil War governor.

LUNCH/DESTINATION OPTIONS ON OR
JUST OFF THE PARKWAY

* Waynesboro, VA
* Tuggle Gap, VA
* Mabry Mill, Meadows of Dan, VA (always a wait to be served)
* Meadows of Dan, VA
* Orchard Gap, VA
* Fancy Gap, VA
* Blowing Rock, NC
* Northwest Trading Post, Glendale, Springs, NC (mostly baked goods and beverages)
* Glendale Springs, NC
* Little Switzerland, NC
* Mount Mitchell State Park, Burnsville, NC
* Asheville, NC
* Cherokee, NC

PART 4
Appendixes

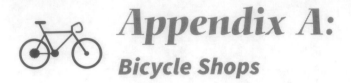

Appendix A:
Bicycle Shops

Though we have already listed bicycle shops in our point-by-point descriptions, we thought a directory organized by city would be helpful for anyone needing a quick reference. As you can see, there are very few bike shops spread out over 570 miles. Some of these shops are a considerable distance or change in elevation from Skyline Drive or the Blue Ridge Parkway. Preventive maintenance is in your best interest. As indicated, a few shops may pick up stranded bicyclists who have major repair problems on the Parkway.

Winchester, Virginia
BLUE RIDGE BICYCLES   540-662-1510;
blueridgebicycles@yahoo.com
> From I-81, take the US 50 exit into town. This turns into Jubal Early Drive. Turn left onto Loudon Street. Go through two traffic lights and look for the shop on the left.
> Monday–Friday, 10 a.m.–6 p.m.; Saturday, 10 a.m.–5 p.m.

ELEMENT SPORTS   540-662-5744; elementsport.com
> From I-81, take the US 50 exit into town. This turns into Jubal Early Drive. Turn left onto Loudon Street. Go through one traffic light and look for the shop on the right.
> 2009 S Loudon St. Monday–Saturday, 9 a.m.–6 p.m.

Waynesboro, Virginia
ROCKFISH GAP OUTFITTERS   540-943-1461;
rockfishgapoutfitters.com
> 1461 E Main St. Monday–Saturday, 10 a.m.–6 p.m.; Sunday, noon–5 p.m.
> Emergency bicycle pickup for major repairs.

Lexington, Virginia

THE LEXINGTON BIKE SHOP   540-463-7969

130 S Main St. Monday–Friday, 9 a.m.–noon and 1–5 p.m.; Saturday, 9 a.m.–noon.

Lynchburg, Virginia

BIKES UNLIMITED CYCLING   434-385-4157; bikesunlimited.com

This shop is 20 miles from the Parkway south on US 501. Estimated time by bicycle on curvy US 501 South into Lynchburg is 1–2 hours, depending on cycling ability.

1312 Jefferson St. Monday–Friday, 10 a.m.–7 p.m.; Saturday, 10 a.m.–5 p.m.

Emergency bicycle pickup for major repairs.

Roanoke, Virginia

CARDINAL BICYCLE   540-344-2453; cardinalbicycle.com

2901 Orange Ave. NE (US 460 East). Monday–Friday, 10 a.m.–7 p.m.; Saturday, 9 a.m.–5 p.m.

EAST COASTERS BIKE SHOP 540-774-7933; eastcoasters.com

3544 Electric Rd., a mile north of Tanglewood Mall. Monday–Friday, 11 a.m.–7 p.m.; Saturday, 10 a.m.–5 p.m.; Sunday, noon–4 p.m.

Emergency bicycle pickup for major repairs.

Boone, North Carolina

BOONE BIKE AND TOURING CO.   828-262-5750; boonebike.com

774 E King St. Monday–Saturday, 10 a.m.–6 p.m.

MAGIC CYCLES INC.   828-265-2211; magiccycles.com

140 S Depot St. #2, behind Farmers Hardware. Monday–Saturday, 10 a.m.–6 p.m.

Emergency bicycle pickup for major repairs.

Asheville, North Carolina

LIBERTY BICYCLES   828-274-2453; libertybikes.com

1378 Hendersonville Rd. Monday–Saturday, 10 a.m.–6 p.m.;
Sunday, noon–5 p.m.

HEARN'S CYCLING & FITNESS   828-253-4800

About 6.8 miles from the Parkway; located downtown.
28 Asheland Ave. Monday–Saturday, 8:30 a.m.–5:30 p.m.

BIOWHEELS   828-236-2453; biowheels.com

About 5.5 miles from the Parkway; located downtown.
81 Coxe Ave. Tuesday–Friday, noon–6 p.m.; Saturday,
noon–5 p.m.

PRO BIKES OF ASHEVILLE   828-253-2800; pro-bikes.com

610 Haywood Rd. Monday–Friday, 10 a.m.–7 p.m.; Saturday,
10 a.m.–5 p.m.; Sunday, 9 a.m.–2 p.m.
Emergency bicycle pickup for major repairs.

SKI COUNTRY SPORTS   828-254-2771; skicountrysports.com

1000 Merrimon Ave. Monday–Saturday, 10 a.m.–6 p.m.
Emergency bicycle pickup for major repairs.

**CAROLINA FATZ CYCLING CENTER   828-665-7744;
carolinafatzmountainbicycle.com**

Follow NC 191 less than 1 mile from the Parkway.
1240 Brevard Rd. #3. Monday–Saturday, 10 a.m.–6 p.m.
Emergency bicycle pickup for major repairs.

Pisgah Forest, North Carolina

**THE HUB AT BACKCOUNTRY OUTDOORS   828-884-8670;
thehubpisgah.com**

Exit 276 South and travel 15 miles to the intersection of US
64. Look for the lizard on the roof. Featuring bikes, outdoor
gear, and beer in the tavern.
Monday–Friday, 10 a.m.–6 p.m.; Saturday, 9 a.m.–6 p.m.;
Sunday, 10 a.m.–5 p.m.

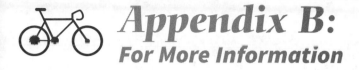

Appendix B:
For More Information

Shenandoah National Park

For maps and information on Skyline Drive and Shenandoah National Park:

540-999-3500; nps.gov/shen

For a brochure listing additional books and maps on Shenandoah National Park:

540-999-3582; snpbooks.org

For a directory of facilities in and surrounding Shenandoah National Park:

Shenandoah Valley Travel Association
877-847-4878; visitshenandoah.org

Blue Ridge Parkway

For maps and information on the Blue Ridge Parkway:

828-298-0398; nps.gov/blri

The Blue Ridge Parkway Association now has an excellent app for smartphones and tablets–Blue Ridge Parkway Travel Planner. Like it on Facebook for up-to-date postings on closures and events on the Parkway. For a directory of facilities along the Blue Ridge Parkway:

Blue Ridge Parkway Association, Inc.
828-271-4779

For information on how to preserve different aspects of the Parkway:

Friends of the Blue Ridge Parkway
800-228-7275; friendsbrp.org

The Blue Ridge Parkway Foundation has raised more than $3.4 million in private funds to support National Park Service projects on the Parkway. If you live in North Carolina, you can purchase a Blue Ridge Parkway license plate; the funds go to the foundation.

Blue Ridge Parkway Foundation
336-721-0260; brpfoundation.org

Smartphone Apps

Blue Ridge Parkway Travel Planner features attractions, lodging, camping, cultural sites, museums, overlooks, history, and shopping.

BRP Tracker is another app that features a map with plotted mile-post points of attraction.

State Tourism Offices

Virginia Tourism Corporation **800-847-4882; virginia.org**

Division of Tourism
North Carolina Department of Commerce
800-847-4862; visitnc.com

Chambers of Commerce and Visitor/Convention Bureaus

NORTH CAROLINA

ASHEVILLE

Asheville Area Chamber of Commerce
828-258-6114; ashevillechamber.org

Asheville Convention & Visitors Bureau
828-258-6101; exploreasheville.com

BANNER ELK

Banner Elk Tourism and Development Authority/Avery County Chamber of Commerce
828-898-5605; banner-elk.com

BLACK MOUNTAIN

Black Mountain–Swannanoa Chamber of Commerce
828-669-2300; 800-669-2301; blackmountain.org

BLOWING ROCK

Blowing Rock Tourism Development Authority
828-295-4636; 877-750-4636; blowingrock.com

BOONE

Watauga County Tourism Development Authority
828-264-1299; 828-266-1345; exploreboonearea.com

BREVARD

Brevard/Transylvania Chamber of Commerce
828-883-3700; 800-648-4523; brevardncchamber.org

BURNSVILLE

Yancey County Chamber of Commerce
828-682-7413; yanceychamber.com

CHEROKEE

Cherokee County Chamber of Commerce
828-837-2242; cherokeecountychamber.com

MAGGIE VALLEY

Maggie Valley Area Visitors Bureau
828-926-1686; 800-624-4431; maggievalley.org

SPARTA

Alleghany Chamber of Commerce
336-372-5473; 800-372-5473; sparta-nc.com

SPRUCE PINE

Mitchell County Chamber of Commerce
828-765-9033; mitchell-county.com

WEST JEFFERSON

Ashe County Chamber of Commerce
336-846-9550; 888-343-2743; ashechamber.com

VIRGINIA

CHARLOTTESVILLE

Charlottesville Regional Chamber of Commerce
434-295-3141; cvillechamber.com

FRONT ROYAL

Front Royal–Warren County Chamber of Commerce
540-635-3185; frontroyalchamber.com

GALAX

Twin County Regional Chamber of Commerce
276-236-2184; twincountychamber.com

LURAY

Luray–Page County Chamber of Commerce
540-743-3915; 888-743-3915; luraypage.com

ROANOKE

Roanoke Regional Chamber of Commerce
540-983-0700 ; roanokechamber.org

The Roanoke Valley Convention and Visitors Bureau
540-342-6025; visitroanokeva.com

STAUNTON AND WAYNESBORO

Greater Augusta Regional Chamber of Commerce
540-324-1133; augustava.com

VINTON

Vinton Area Chamber of Commerce
540-343-1364; vintonchamber.com

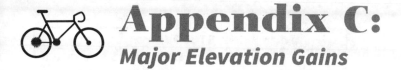

Appendix C:
Major Elevation Gains

This data, compiled by Tom DeVaughn of Troutville, Virginia, provides you with a quick tally of the gains in elevation along the Blue Ridge Parkway. The chart does two things: it divides the Parkway into sections and adds up the total number of feet climbed within sections. It also specifies at what mileposts major uphills begin and end, with the elevation climbed for each uphill. For example, southbound between Mileposts 4.7 and 8.5, the Parkway has a continuous gain in elevation of 1,100 feet.

Note: Beginning a ride at 3,000 feet and cycling to 4,500 feet does not mean a simple gain of 1,500 feet. Skyline Drive and the Parkway both rise and fall any number of times before arriving at certain elevations. You may climb the same 500 feet four or five times without any indication on National Park Service maps.

While we provide this chart and the elevation profile graphs in the point-by-point descriptions, we hope that you will not be intimidated by elevation. Try not to dwell on the task. Just take in the scenery and enjoy the subtle changes each 500 feet can make.

NORTHBOUND			
MILEPOSTS	TOTAL ELEV. CLIMBED	MAJOR UPHILLS MILEPOSTS	ELEVATION CHANGE
0–24	1,450 ft.	13.7–10.7	563 ft.
		9.2–8.5	222 ft.
		4.7–3.0	300 ft.
24.0–48.0	2,670 ft.	46.4–43.9	627 ft.
		40.0–38.8	331 ft.
		37.4–34.0	951 ft.
48.0–63.0	1,870 ft.	63.0–49.3	1,852 ft.
63.0–76.7	0 ft.		3,305 ft.
76.7–96.0	2,865 ft.	93.1–91.6	374 ft.
		89.1–87.3	634 ft.
		85.6–84.7	230 ft.
		83.5–76.7	1,490 ft.
96.0–120.4	2,680 ft.	115.0–113.0	280 ft.
		106.0–103.6	500 ft.
		102.5–99.8	820 ft.
120.4	Mill Mountain Spur—length to summit: 3.1 miles. Elevation climbed from Parkway to summit: 580 ft.; elevation climbed from summit to Parkway: 330 ft.		
120.4–144.0	2,006 ft.	140.1–139.3	229 ft.
		136.0–134.9	285 ft.
		124.6–123.1	320 ft.
		121.4–120.4	265 ft.
144.0–168.0	1,840 ft.	159.4–157.6	389 ft.
		150.6–149.8	226 ft.
168.0–192.0	2,445 ft.	189.4–188.7	220 ft.
		175.1–171.9	575 ft.
		168.9–168.0	185 ft.
192.0–216.0	2,225 ft.	215.6–214.0	260 ft.
		210.6–209.4	222 ft.
		199.4–198.7	165 ft.
216.0–240.0	1,566 ft.	240.0–239.3	160 ft.
		238.5–237.2	270 ft.
		220.8–220.1	205 ft.
240.0–264.6	2,625 ft.	257.8–256.8	200 ft.
		248.0–244.5	495 ft.
		243.8–242.9	270 ft.
		242.4–241.5	300 ft.
264.6–288.0	3,050 ft.	285.2–283.8	400 ft.

SOUTHBOUND			
MILEPOSTS	**TOTAL ELEV. CLIMBED**	**MAJOR UPHILLS MILEPOSTS**	**ELEVATION CHANGE**
0–24	2,810 ft.	0–3	391 ft.
		4.7–8.5	1,100 ft.
		9.2–10.7	322 ft.
		18.5–23.0	785 ft.
24.0–48.0	1,742 ft.	37.4–38.8	229 ft.
		42.0–43.9	570 ft.
		47.0–48.0	177 ft.
48.0–63.0	250 ft.	48.0–49.3	228 ft.
63.0–76.7	3,305 ft.	63.0–76.7	3,305 ft.
76.7–96.0	1,360 ft.	89.1–91.6	569 ft.
		93.1–95.4	428 ft.
96.0–120.4	1,657 ft.	118.1–120.4	462 ft.
120.4	Mill Mountain Spur—length to summit: 3.1 miles. Elevation climbed from Parkway to summit: 580 ft.; elevation climbed from summit to Parkway: 330 ft.		
120.4–144.0	3,200 ft.	127.0–132.5	1,400 ft.
		134.0–134.9	195 ft.
		136.4–138.2	275 ft.
144.0–168.0	2,530 ft.	150.6–152.1	278 ft.
		157.0–157.6	200 ft.
		164.7–168.0	830 ft.
168.0–192.0	1,745 ft.	169.5–170.1	260 ft.
		176.2–177.0	212 ft.
		186.6–188.8	360 ft.
192.0–216.0	2,047 ft.	195.0–196.2	235 ft.
		197.6–198.7	210 ft.
		200.5–201.5	335 ft.
216.0–240.0	2,530 ft.	216.6–217.7	240 ft.
		231.3–233.1	550 ft.
		233.7–235.2	280 ft.
		235.8–236.9	365 ft.
240.0–264.6	2,680 ft.	240.0–240.8	170 ft.
		249.0–249.8	235 ft.
		251.3–252.8	300 ft.
		263.6–264.6	360 ft.
264.6–288.0	3,160 ft.	265.2–266.8	270 ft.

NORTHBOUND			
MILEPOSTS	TOTAL ELEV. CLIMBED	MAJOR UPHILLS MILEPOSTS	ELEVATION CHANGE
		279.6–278.8	270 ft.
		276.4–273.1	910 ft.
		269.8–268.6	315 ft.
		268.1–266.8	380 ft.
288.0–312.0	2,185 ft.	309.9–306.5	460 ft.
		305.6–305.0	200 ft.
		295.8–293.8	555 ft.
		291.8–289.9	275 ft.
312.0–336.3	3,120 ft.	336.3–335.7	215 ft.
		327.4–325.8	290 ft.
		325.0–320.7	1,210 ft.
		316.4–312.4	520 ft.
336.3–358.5	1,705 ft.	351.9–349.9	565 ft.
		334.1–341.8	530 ft.
		339.8–338.9	260 ft.
355.4	Spur Road to Mount Mitchell is 4.8 miles in length. Total elevation climbed from Parkway is 1,390 ft.		
358.5–384.0	4,265 ft.	383.5–376.7	1,135 ft.
		375.3–364.1	2,535 ft.
		361.1–358.5	540 ft.
384.0–408.0	850 ft.	none	3,705 ft.
408.0–431.4	1,835 ft.	426.5–424.8	325 ft.
(431.4 is the Parkway's highest elevation)		423.2–421.6	250 ft.
		415.6–413.2	385 ft.
		411.9–409.6	400 ft.
431.4–469.1	7,470 ft.	469.1–462.2	2,240 ft.
		461.6–458.9	1,000 ft.
		455.7–451.2	1,480 ft.
		443.1–435.5	2,020 ft.
		433.3–431.4	475 ft.
458.2 Spur road	Heintooga to Balsam Mtn.		
		3.6–1.0	860 ft.
		Total Uphill Climb North: 48,722 ft.	

SOUTHBOUND			
MILEPOSTS	TOTAL ELEV. CLIMBED	MAJOR UPHILLS MILEPOSTS	ELEVATION CHANGE
		269.8–271.1	330 ft.
		271.4–273.1	575 ft.
		276.4–277.4	375 ft.
		281.7–282.4	280 ft.
		282.7–283.8	255 ft.
		286.0–287.8	500 ft.
288.0–312.0	2,210 ft.	288.7–289.9	250 ft.
		291.8–293.8	400 ft.
		298.6–302.1	1,005 ft.
312.0–336.3	2,705 ft.	316.4–318.2	380 ft.
		318.5–320.7	590 ft.
		330.9–332.1	410 ft.
		332.6–334.5	545 ft.
336.3–358.5	4,060 ft.	336.3–338.9	540 ft.
		345.4–349.9	1,480 ft.
		351.9–355.0	920 ft.
		355.4–358.5	520 ft.
355.4	Spur Road to Mount Mitchell is 4.8 miles in length. Total elevation climbed from Parkway is 1,390 ft.		
358.5–384.0	680 ft.	361.1–364.1	500 ft.
384.0–408.0		393.8–396.4	920 ft.
		397.3–399.7	430 ft.
		400.3–405.5	965 ft.
		405.7–407.7	745 ft.
408.0–431.4	2,775 ft.	416.8–420.2	1,100 ft.
(431.4 is the		423.2–424.8	230 ft.
Parkway's high-		426.5–428.2	405 ft.
est elevation)		429.0–431.4	600 ft.
431.4–469.1	3,450 ft.	443.1–451.2	2,450 ft.
		455.7–458.9	810 ft.
458.2	Heintooga to Balsam Mtn.		
Spur road		0.0–1.0	255 ft.
		3.6–8.6	845 ft.
Total Uphill Climb South: 48,601 ft.			

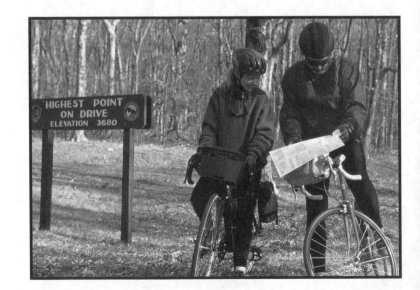

Two cyclists stop to confer with their map just before reaching Skyland Resort.

Index

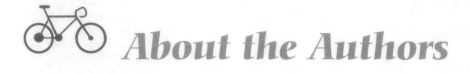

About the Authors

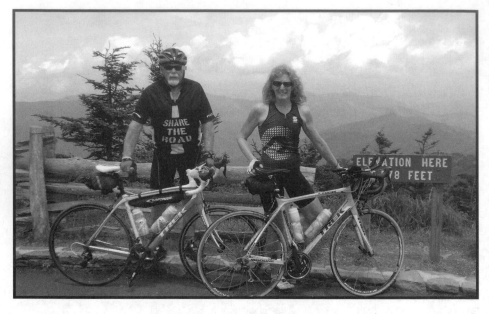

Libby and Charlie Skinner at Mount Mitchell, North Carolina

Libby and Charlie Skinner moved to North Carolina from Jacksonville, Florida, in 1985 and have been bicycling the Blue Ridge Parkway and Skyline Drive for nearly 30 years. They have cycled Skyline Drive and the Blue Ridge Parkway end-to-end several times and have toured throughout the western and southeastern United States. They are also the authors of *The Best Bike Rides in the South*, 2nd edition (Globe Pequot Press, 1996).

The Skinners live in Winston-Salem, North Carolina, where Libby is the assistant director of the Forsyth County Public Library, and Charlie, who is retired, can cycle whenever he wants. Libby also competes in triathlons and enjoys swimming and running almost as much as her first love–cycling. The Skinners have three daughters: Bonnie, Caroline, and Katie.